YOUNG LIVING

Escaping Diabetes Through Healthy Living

Cora Parker

ISBN: 979-8-9873546-0-5

Front cover and book design by Carol Noon.

First printing, 2023

coraparker.com

DEDICATION

I dedicate this book to my beloved husband who makes things happen, my children and their wives for conquering all challenges, my precious grandchildren who keep me on my toes, my sisters, and their families, and to my family that live in the Philippines that make my life exciting. I also dedicate this book to Angie Neff, Mary Chambers and Tess Thomas.

Araullo High School Batch `68, this is for you. Cheers!

I thank our Lord Jesus for blessing us with more time to enjoy life and love one another. May we have a lot more good memories to celebrate together.

ACKNOWLEDGEMENT

I am thankful and grateful to our Lord Jesus Christ for giving me the opportunity to write this book, "Young Living".

I am grateful for my husband's contributions, his support, and understanding the whole time I have been writing.

I cannot express enough gratitude to my editors, Sarah Parker and Carol Noon for their committed support. I would never have gotten this book going without their skill and precision.

I am grateful to my mentor, Andrew Zollman, for strengthening my knowledge in writing a book and Lourdes Rose for her help and guidance.

Thank you to my sons for encouraging me to write. Thank you to everyone in my "Writer's Utopia" group who helped me get this book started. JA (Julie), Rebecca Fonseca, Jean Dunstan, Rob Mata, and special thanks to JL Lahey for his constructive advice. I would also like to acknowledge Vanessa Knizley, who has told me wise things about how to improve my writing. I would never have got my work in the right direction without her vision. She is such a blessing. Thankful to Jenifer LeRoy, Katleen Chernek, Kelly Hotel, Jose S. Lisa Mier and Chris Avelar for their support and contributions. I appreciate Janalyn Buseck, Jen Nacis and Shannon Fenzel for their contributions.

Finally, I am grateful for my family members Kerri Parker, Aiden and Ava Parker, Mikael Wolfert, Makhiba Williams, Rebecca Tyynismaa, Violeta Johnson, Stacey Busey, Jamie and Jean Noon for their support and contributions.

TABLE OF CONTENTS

PREFACE

This book was inspired by the disease that my family has suffered and died from. Escaping diabetes through healthy living was possible, for me, through healthy living. I was diagnosed pre-diabetic a few years ago. I was able to change my daily habits, and through healthy living I have escaped diabetes. I am happy and live a fulfilled life at 72. My prayer is that healthy living may keep me and everybody around me healthy. This book will serve to encourage myself and others to live healthier lives.

Healthy living will inspire us to keep the unhealthy habits at bay. It will encourage us to make better choices and decisions for ourselves. Prioritizing health is beneficial for everybody. Life is awesome and beautiful with healthy living. I can enjoy the things I want to do with friends and family. Life turns ugly very fast when loved ones become ill and I hate to see them battle their illnesses. Watching my family members suffer, and some who have died due to complications resulting from diabetes, is what inspired me to write this book, "Young Living".

I am not a doctor nor a healthcare provider, but I am a teacher. What I am sharing in this book comes from my own experience, research, interviews, and conversations with family, friends, acquaintances, and even strangers. I have learned so much, but there is still much to learn.

"I can do all things through him who strengthens me." - Philippians 4:13

I will continue to work on healthy living until our Lord takes me home. I have no desire to live forever, I just want to enjoy the time that I have left. I want to encourage as many people as possible to take good care of their health. Doing research, and interviewing family, friends, and strangers, as well as reading and writing was exhausting, but in the end, I found it to be quite exciting. Now I know that for me, there is no place for boredom. I love learning and am excited to share with the world my passion and knowledge for healthy living.

"For I know the thoughts that I think toward you, says the LORD, thoughts of peace and not of evil, to give you a future and a hope." - Jeremiah 29:11

This verse means God wants us to succeed, and I am confident that our Lord will be with us on this journey. "Young Living", Part I will focus on the 7 essentials for healthy living. Part II How stress has affected me and could possibly affect others. Part III includes my personal nutrition and supplements that I use to escape diabetes.

INTRODUCTION

Young Living" is living with a positive attitude. Young living happens when a person is youthful, selfless, enthusiastic, lively, blooming, refreshed, and energetic. This person enjoys life to the fullest, loves life, is outgoing, and is vigorous in achieving their goals. They have vitality and continue to grow physically, mentally, socially, and spiritually. Young living is healthy living. Young living has less inflammation, fewer doctor's visits, and may live longer than their older-feeling peers. When I get sick, I bounce right back. I was diagnosed as pre-diabetic a few years ago. I escaped diabetes through healthy living. Occasionally, people with diabetes at an early stage of the disease improve their health through healthy living. Full-blown diabetics may manage their condition through healthy living.

Spiritual vitality, mindfulness, and positive thinking play a significant role in young living. The easiest way to get rid of negativity is to speak positively. This book is focused on type 2 diabetes which my family and friends have suffered and died from. For now, it has been possible for me to escape diabetes through healthy living. My prayer is that healthy living may keep me and everybody healthy. This book, "Young Living," will encourage others to live healthier lives. Change has helped me in so many ways. I now keep going forward. What can I create today? What can I do to help? It just keeps my spirit free. I love it. Healthy living is the best way of life. It increases energy and allows for a fruitful, fulfilled, happier life.

My mom passed away in her forties, and my three younger siblings have died before me because of diabetes. I was terrified when my youngest brother died in January of 2022. He was a slave of pleasure. He partied and went to the casino, even while he was on dialysis! He was scheduled for amputation but died of sepsis before they could do the procedure. He spent his last six months in misery. All his life, he just wanted to have fun. I wonder, though, did he truly have fun? He might not have died at such a young age if only he had cared better for himself and made better choices.

As I have been blessed throughout my 72 years of life, I want to pay it forward and pass these pearls of wisdom on to others. I am excited to share the knowledge I have gained from my experiences, research, and interviews that I have done. One evening, I sat on her living room floor with my neighbor Jennifer, who is 57 years old. We were there for quite some time, conversing and catching up on life. When it was time for us to get up, Jennifer exclaimed, "Cora, I swear you look and move like you are at least forty years younger than you are!" I was already standing there as she was struggling to get up. She first asked me to help her. She said that her right leg had fallen asleep, and her final complaint was how much her hips were hurting her. The reason why she wanted me to share this with you is because she admires my attitude toward life and my uplifting personality. She wanted you to know how much she values what I feel I must share.

If we are happy, we are healthy. My research taught me about hormones and endorphins that contribute to our happiness. They are natural painkillers. Eating my favorite food will make me happy, but I watch my portions and eat in moderation. I do things that make me happy and have a good time.   More on happy hormones in Chapter X.

According to the World Health Organization (WHO), self-care is important because it can help promote health, prevent disease, and help individuals, families, and communities promote health and cope with illness and disabilities. Self-care can be accomplished with and without the support of a healthcare provider. We will discuss more on self-care in Chapter II.

Love you guys! See you in Part I.

Part I:
7 ESSENTIALS FOR HEALTHY LIVING

CHAPTER I:
The Power of Planning and Having a Routine

There are a lot of things we can do to impact our health and quality of life. We already *know* that making healthy choices can help us feel better and be more beneficial, but we must also act on this knowledge and desire to change our lives. It can be frustrating to experience setbacks when trying to make changes to reach a goal related to our health, but the good news is it can impact our habits now and in the future.

Planning and Cognitive Theory

Always start by planning the day. A plan is essential for productivity. Without a plan for the day, the only thing moving will be fingers on the remote and a few steps to the refrigerator and pantry. Then back to warming up the couch and becoming a couch potato. This is a good recipe for boredom and diabetes. Let this go on too long, and then life will switch from boredom to treating diabetes. It doesn't have to be this way—just plan.

I start the day by planning to improve myself and my self-care. I make myself the priority. Every day the plan should include something to maintain good health. Get up, do some stretching, and learn something new. Go out, get some sun and fresh air. Call Mom or a friend you haven't seen in a long time.

I'll be honest with you; I did not want to go to the gym today. Then, I worked on changing the format and sections of my book. The section I was shuffling said, "fifteen minutes of exercise is beneficial to your health." Great! Now I have to go! You see, even I struggle to keep up with this idea. A glance at the clock, and it is already bedtime. Today is gone, and it is not coming back. Focus is easier when your desire is strong enough to accomplish your goals. Focus, focus, focus.

In short, a plan helps us to:

- **Set direction and priorities:** A plan helps us know what we should be working on and what we should work on first. It also helps to simplify decision-making and prioritize the activities necessary for success.

- **Drive Alignment:** When we have a plan for the day or a task, it helps us to get everyone on the same page and move together to achieve the goal and desired outcome. It helps to develop a strategy that serves as the vehicle to align all resources and maximize success.

- **Communicate the message and end goal:** When everyone knows what each person is doing, it allows more significant opportunities for people to maximize success.

It isn't easy when starting out, but as we see progress, we are inspired and enjoy it. We must stay focused and pass that stage where we are challenged.

Cognitive Theory is the ideology that attempts to define and explain human behavior by studying the mental processes involved in developing and comprehending thoughts and actions. Cognition is the mental state and method of gaining knowledge and understanding through thought, senses, and experiences. It includes conscious and unconscious processes such as perception, recognition, conceiving, and reasoning. While there are many aspects of cognition, psychologists typically look at cognitive processes because they affect learning and behavior.

Swiss psychologist Jean Piaget viewed cognition as an adaptation of two basic processes: assimilation and accommodation. First, let's talk about assimilation. Piaget states that assimilation is the process of how a person interprets reality in terms of their internal model of the world (based on previous experience). On the other hand, Piaget defined accommodation as a representation of the changes a person makes to their model of the world through the process of adjusting to experience.

An American psychologist, Jerome Bruner, took Piaget's theory further and suggested that cognitive processes are impacted by three conditions used to represent the world. First, is the enactive mode, which is representation through action. Second is the iconic mode, which uses visual and mental images, and the third is the symbolic mode, which uses language.

In essence, the theory of cognitive thinking means what I think impacts what I believe, which affects what I do. Life is a choice. We either choose to live or die. I remember that old saying, "An empty mind is a devil's workshop." I am bored when I am not doing anything, and life becomes dull and worthless. I start to deteriorate.

The other side of the coin is that if I am enjoying what I am doing, then I keep doing it, and that makes me happier. There are also a lot of temptations that will cross my mind: eating unhealthy foods, doing something I will regret later, or going somewhere I am not supposed to be. I am careful about how and what I think because my life is shaped by my thoughts.

Choosing Wholesome Activities

My granddaughter made a comment after she read my rough draft. She said, "Lola, I am not going to watch too much TV anymore and start doing things

I've wanted to do for a long time. I am going to have a fun-filled life." (Lola is what we say for "grandma" in the Philippines.)

I always have a choice. Bored? I can't let time pass me by. Today will not come back. Let's be thankful and make the best of it. Learn something new every day. It is fun, stimulates our minds and body, and helps us make better decisions and choices. Learning improves our knowledge, and we become confident in all areas of life. We start to build confidence in doing things we normally wouldn't. We begin to look forward to what the day will bring.

When I choose wholesome activities for my day, I appreciate life and enjoy it. On the other hand, if I just lay around and do nothing, then I become bored. I make my own decisions and choices; I can't blame my situations on others.

Plan to Enjoy the Power of Sunshine

The first rays of morning sunlight stimulate serotonin and cortisol production. This gently awakens us from our slumber. Then, sunlight detected via the retina throughout our day prompts the release of more serotonin which regulates appetite and calms our mood. The onset of darkness drives the conversion of serotonin into sleep-inducing melatonin. Leaving the curtains open to allow the morning sunlight in and avoiding electronic screens at night can help improve sleep patterns. This can also ensure that we awake feeling refreshed.

The sun is also a key ingredient in vitamin D production. Having healthy levels of vitamin D is associated with a brighter mood. Studies have also shown, however, that getting plenty of exposure to the sun can reduce depression and fatigue - regardless of vitamin D levels.

You are not alone if you feel gloomy or down in the winter! Seasonal Affective Disorder is a type of depression that arises with the changing seasons. This occurs most often when less sunlight occurs in the winter months. Sun exposure enables the production of hormones that reduce stress, block pain, and protect heart health. Sun exposure also aids in producing beta-endorphins, which have opiate-like effects on the brain and may be addictive. This often results in withdrawal-like effects when sun exposure is reduced.

Vitamin D, often called the "Sunshine Vitamin," is a fat-soluble nutrient that prompts the immune system to fight infections. It is also essential for intestinal calcium absorption and regulating calcium levels in the blood. Vitamin D deficiency can cause several health issues including insomnia, seasonal affective disorder, heart issues, gut dysfunction, softening of the teeth and bones, and even slow physical development in infants and children.

The signs and symptoms of Vitamin D deficiency include nervousness, diarrhea, burning in the mouth and throat, nearsightedness, muscle weakness, and cramping. Elevated follicle-stimulating hormones, iron deficiency, increased serum phosphate, and high parathyroid hormone levels often accompany vitamin D deficiency.

We should spend at least thirty minutes per day in the sun (with arms or legs exposed, at minimum) to ensure we're getting enough vitamin D. Sunshine is essential for our health, but everything is in moderation. Too much sun will cause sunburn and a greater risk of skin cancer. I take advantage of the morning sunshine. It always rejuvenates me and makes me feel energetic. Go outside, enjoy the fresh air and the power of sunshine.

Escaping Diabetes Through Healthy Living

Right now, I have no medication, love learning, reading, writing, and watching comedy and inspiring movies. I am healthy, loving, caring, enthusiastic, and optimistic. I took Home Economics at the University of Central Missouri, Warrensburg, Missouri. I graduated in 1984 but am guilty because I don't like to cook and cannot sew. My strengths are in Family Living and Family Development, and because of this, I learned about nutrition early on.

Staying fit physically

To stay fit physically, I go to the gym. I accomplish two short-term goals when I go to the gym: exercise and social interaction for a healthy lifestyle. They offer wonderful classes at the gym, and most of the time, I don't even notice that I have already finished an hour of exercise. I can't do that at home because there are too many distractions. I'll be following someone on YouTube, and after five minutes, I'll be gardening, then vacuuming or playing with my dog.

Another benefit of going to the gym is visiting with my friends before and after classes. It is fun and fills my social meter. Sometimes, we even go for coffee together afterward. This time is fun and relaxing for me. Going to those classes at the gym also gives me an excuse to go somewhere and to leave the house. It is also something scheduled which provides structure to my day. Afterward, I go back home and eat a healthy meal. My short-term goals of a healthy lifestyle, diet, and exercise are done for the day. Mission accomplished!

Staying fit socially

Remember in the olden days when children played outside, ran, climbed a tree, played hide and seek, played ball, and so on? Nowadays, children play games on their devices instead of with family or friends. They have become isolated. Many of them hardly participate in any physical activities. Not all of them; there are still some, very few, it seems, that are healthy and notice and care about their health.

I realized this same concept of isolation was part of the reason I became bored and lonely. I need to socialize and be around people, so I go to the gym to socialize while also exercising. The same goes for learning. It is so easy to Google everything when we have a question or want to look something up, but then we lose out on interacting with others, like when going to the library or attending a class or seminar. I discovered that I love the Yuma Main Library. The staff is very helpful to all patrons, from the youngest to the seniors. They are so friendly and walk me through everything I need to learn. I have learned so much since I started writing. It's amazing! If you want to learn something new, start with your local library - you'll be glad you did!

Remember the saying, "No man is an island." This saying comes from a sermon by seventeenth-century English author John Donne. It means no one is self-sufficient, and everyone relies on others. This is very true for me. I had a lot of help writing this book. I received a lot of good advice, and a few were not interested, but I am thankful for the blessings and the joy of writing and making new friends in the process.

Staying fit mentally and emotionally

Not only do we have to stay fit physically, but we must also stay fit mentally and emotionally. For myself, I have chosen writing to help keep healthy mentally and emotionally. When I retired ten years ago, I was miserable. I didn't know what to do with my time and never had any plans. I read many books on happiness for years, but nothing ever came from it. It seemed like a waste of time. Then, I realized enjoying what I am doing solves my problem. That's it! Enjoying what we are doing will make us happy.

When my youngest brother died at the beginning of 2022, I started searching for what I enjoyed doing. I finally discovered that it was writing. It excites me so much that I finish my chores quickly so I can go back to writing. My hard work and research to make myself and others become better people, happier, fulfilled and making better choices help me with my mental and emotional well-being. My interest in writing the book even improved my outlook on life. My relationship with my husband and understanding of the people around me also improved. That alone is a significant payback for writing this book.

When I decided to write this book, I already felt young. While working on it, I feel even more youthful. When my friends give me ideas, I jump on them. I have been researching, learning, interviewing, and discovering how other people care for themselves and what they eat. I felt sad that most people still drink a lot of soda (and not only drinking soda, but they are super-sized sodas), eat a lot of junk food, and are hardly moving at all. Some people get help from the government or family members just to survive. Many are unaware that their lifestyle may lead to diabetes or other health conditions. Many people I talked to sounded unhappy, irritable, bored, and cranky.

I was irritable and cranky too. It was boring when I did not have any plan or direction. Being unhappy is not fun. My husband and I fought about nonsense just for something to do for a long time. We solved our issues without trying to solve them. It was not on my list to fix our relationship. The way I saw it, nothing was wrong with me; he was the problem. Boredom made me miserable. Then, a miracle happened!

I didn't find out until I started writing that I always feel inspired. Unfortunately, it's not one size fits all. Writing brings me so much joy, but it may not work for everyone. When I started writing, my whole life began to make sense. Remember, I was just bored. My routine had become the same thing on different days. It was awful. Now, I wake up refreshed, excited, and happy with what the day will bring. It does make all the difference when I have something planned. Waking up and expecting the day to go well will not happen if I don't plan anything. It's fun to live with my husband again! It wasn't him; it was me who was hard to live with. This taught me not to assume the other person is the only one with the problem. It is best to look at myself first. My attitudes are affecting our marriage and our health.

When I am in a bad mood, my health goes bad too. That's what happened to us. In the past, I've had to have carbs or sugar to make me feel better. Even worse, I would eat bigger portions to fill that empty gap. I think clearly now, and I make better choices. I am doing what makes me happy. Doing something that I like will bring me joy, and I am fulfilled. It was a rude awakening and wasn't a good feeling, but now life is fun again!

Staying fit spiritually

Meditation, praying, and writing in my gratitude and thankfulness journals are ways I stay fit spiritually. For me, to remain young and healthy, I must believe in God. I must keep God within me, for He is the "Light," the "Love," and the "Life." He lights the right of faith as gratitude for what we haven't seen or experienced yet. Hebrews 11:1 (NKJV) says, *"Now faith is the substance of things hoped for the evidence of things not seen."* It takes faith to be thankful for what we cannot see and have not yet experienced, but this is how miracles happen.

Health is a complex issue. Not everyone is healthy; some are going through dialysis, high blood pressure, mental illness, heart disease, stroke, boredom, diabetes, depression, cancer, and more. I feel your pain. I went through boredom, misery, and feeling lost after retiring. At the same time, I was going through a phase where I prayed for peace and joy, but I was still miserable. At that time, we were eating out all the time, and we traveled a lot, but still, something was not right. Even though I was praying, my faith was tested, and my attitude became terrible. This affected my husband too, and he became angry at me all the time. Through my research, I found out that my attitude made him mad. Now I am working on myself and the strength of my faith.

I pray anywhere where I can communicate easily with God. Jesus is my Lord, Savior, and protector; I ask for his forgiveness daily. He is the only one who is quick to forgive me. I pray for the whole world, for God to watch over my family, friends, and whatever I do. He is an awesome God.

Now, I have peace in my heart and at home. I am at peace wherever I am. I can feel God's presence now and the joy I had before. When times are tough, we should not be discouraged. We all go through rough patches from time to time. Have faith and keep living your dreams. Things will change; nothing lasts forever. Life is boring without something to look forward to, so don't give up, keep working at it. Keep dreaming.

Enjoying Happy Thoughts

Growing up in the Philippines is a pleasant memory for me. There were a lot of fun things that we enjoyed. We had all kinds of celebrations and fiestas for birthdays and holidays. The most memorable was Christmas, Easter, and All Saints Day. My parents would send us to church on- church days, especially Sunday, but my parents didn't go. They just knew there was something good that would happen if we went.

My mom always sewed nice outfits for us for the holidays and special occasions. After church, when there was a celebration, my twin sister and I would rush down to the piñata and gather as much candy as we could. We always got in trouble because our new outfits would be all torn up. My mom still sewed nice outfits for all celebrations, and we kept going home with torn-up clothes from having fun. Sometimes we would get spanked, but it was always worth it. Birthdays and weddings were fun too. All the adults were so busy that we kids got away with a lot of fun because the adults didn't have time for discipline. We took advantage of these opportunities.

In the Philippines, we had the most joyful and longest Christmas celebration that I have ever seen in my whole life. We start to celebrate Christmas when the month starts ending with "ber." We start hanging up the Christmas decorations in September, and the street vendors start selling Christmas foods. Caroling begins on the 16th of December. We would go house to house with homemade instruments and sing Christmas carols. The neighbors would pay us for singing. We would eat good food from home and around our neighborhood. We would also get invited to visit our friends and families all over the place. Our parents would just let us loose. We had a good time.

It is important to pick those good memories to think about once in a while. Good memories bring joy. I live by and enjoy what I am doing and what I have today. The past is gone, and tomorrow is a mystery. The future's not ours to see; let it be. Happiness is a choice. A strong desire always succeeds. When we are determined, we are unstoppable.

When I wake up, I smile and thank God for the good day ahead. I smile before I pick up and answer the phone. This puts my mood in better spirits. When I leave my house and see my neighbor, I smile at my neighbor; this will make me a better neighbor and might brighten their day. I smile at the cashier when they are ringing up my groceries. I smile with my co-workers when I arrive at work. Just remember, smile, smile, smile. I used to make a big deal about nothing. Now, I must let it go. Life is not perfect, and it would be boring if it were. I love challenges!

Loving Others

Let's talk about love. I love this subject. Galatians 5:14 (NIV) says, "Love your neighbor as you love yourself." I don't know when times changed, but I remember the days when we saw somebody walking or needed a ride, and we felt safe to offer a ride. Nowadays, I am suspicious of people around me. If I offer somebody a ride, he'll be the one driving, and I'll be the one walking.

In the 70s, when I was in my twenties, I remember caring for our elders. Family ties were different then. There was always one family member that took care of everybody. Everyone else depended on that one family member. Now, times have changed, and some parents take care of their adult children forever. If you belong to this group, don't get mad at me. It's time to let your parents know how much you love and care for them. Let them know how much you appreciate them before it is too late to let them know. Let your parents know you are there for them as much as they are there for you. That's how we should take care of each other.

I remember getting a lot of spankings, but I still loved my parents. People seem to enjoy others when they are cheerful and loving, but we enjoy their company. Our values have changed, and we focus more on things than our loved ones. The more things I have, the more things I want. The downside is that I am still miserable after acquiring all those things. I stopped chasing things because I won't find joy in them. I can't hug them, love them, or talk to them. Things add clutter to my pleasant life. If I want to be happy, I open my heart and pay more attention to my loved ones than my things. I am thankful for our family, starting from our Father in Heaven.

I am enjoying life, married for almost 50 years now. I met my husband in Angeles City, Philippines, by accident (the details will be in my next book). We have two sons, both of whom are in the military. I'm laughing now because when they were growing up, they both said they'd never join the military; both are now past retirement but still serving. Our grandchildren are all grown up.

The combination of two cultures was, and is, very exciting for my husband and me. There were a lot of learnings and exciting experiences. There was also a lot of frustration, disappointment, and wrong expectations. Marriage is like that: sometimes it is fun, sometimes it is not. I am blessed with a good man. He's not always nice, but he is good. He tries, and that's what matters. I try to remember that even Jesus lost his temper when he was a man.

Example 1

12 Jesus entered the temple courts and drove out all who were buying and selling there. He overturned the tables of the money changers and the benches of those selling doves. 13 "It is written," he said to them, "My house will be called a house of prayer," but you are making it 'a den of robbers'. Matthew 21:12-13 (NIV)

Example 2

22 One day Jesus said to his disciples, "Let us go over to the other side of the lake." So, they got into a boat and set out. 23 As they sailed, he fell asleep. A squall came down on the lake, so that the boat was being swamped, and they were in great danger.24 The disciples went and woke him, saying, "Master, Master, we're going to drown!" He got up and rebuked the wind and the raging waters; the storm subsided, and all was calm. 25 "Where is your faith?" he asked his disciples. In fear and amazement, they asked one another, "Who is this? He commands even the winds and the water, and they obey him." - Luke 8:22-25 (NIV)

God is always with us. Invite him in, and we are never alone. He protects us, our loved ones, and our dreams. He also blesses what we are doing. Believe! Put trust in our Lord Jesus. Psalm 144:15 (KJV) says, *"Happy are the people whose God is the Lord."* God wants us to be happy.

Looking back now, life is kind of like a marriage. They both have ups and downs. The ups were fun, but I also appreciate those downs. The downs made me who I have become; motivated, inspired, happier, stronger, and braver. Now I know I must go through those tough times optimistic and thankful. I am grateful that I passed the tests through all those downs. Pray, pray, pray. Prayer works all the time.

The point is I must look for the best in every situation. I must be the better half, appreciate my blessings, and be understanding and loving to others. I can't be the judgmental one. I cannot just love them when they love me. I have to be better than that. To love is a choice we make. I must choose to love my loved ones no matter what. This will improve my relationships and make me happier and feel better. Love conquers all.

I've also learned that it is hard on my heart when I am angry or frustrated. My heart works twice as much when I am disappointed, frustrated, unhappy, or angry. That's dangerous, and I am not a doormat. I just stay calm and address the issue, not the other person. Let's also talk about finances. That's part of where my anger, frustration, and unhappiness were coming from. Simple living is not there anymore. I spent the money I didn't have and became frustrated because I couldn't save as much as I needed to. This cycle causes stress and frustration. Instead of loving on my loved ones, they became my outlet. I became irritable because things were not going how I wanted them to. Now, I cannot change the past or the future. The past is already gone, and the future is a mystery.

Worry is not alone; it always accompanies impatience. I must live in the present and trust in the Lord. We can find contentment with what we have if we focus on the loving and kind people we are and find joy in our present situation. Reach out to others using our blessings and gifts. There is always something beautiful to talk about. Life is a journey where we can enjoy the scenery, the love, and the blessings each day brings.

The most significant change that has happened is a shift in our values. People don't care and don't think before they act. For many people, they don't care if their actions will harm others. Hurt is not the same as harm. Hurt is a part of life. When we react to our loved ones in a hurtful way, we end up harming them. Instead of getting angry with them, we should put our arms around them, ask if everything is alright, and see what happens. I can't just love them when they love me and then be mean to them when they are mean to me. That's sad. Relationships need unconditional love. When I mistreat my friends or family, I hurt them emotionally. I don't want that. That's why I must love myself because I can't give love I don't have.

My Daily Routine

I want to share my daily routine because some friends I showed my project told me they don't want to read the whole book. Instead, they are only interested in how I stayed in shape. I am warning you, though, if you don't read the entire book, you'll miss a lot. I have also inserted some of my personal secrets throughout the book, including *ancient Filipino secrets.* This section is only the tip of the iceberg!

So, here it is…my daily routine starts in the morning. When I get up, I say my prayer, do my meditation, and log in to my thankful and grateful journal. I sip 2 tsp. of MCT oil with a glass of warm water. I drink up to 2 cups of water if I am thirsty. (I switch to olive oil for a month, then continue my daily routine with MCT oil.). I go outside for at least 15 minutes to get some sun, but it is usually longer. I either work in the garden or clean up outside. I eat breakfast with two eggs, a cup of green tea, a cup of Hershey's Special Dark Chocolate, and two pieces of Ezekiel toast bread.

I enjoy working in the garden, especially in the morning, before I go to the gym. Cutting those big trees gives me muscle. When an old woman has muscle, you know she's physically fit! After working in the garden, I go in and take a shower. Now I have a choice: I can go to the gym or work on my book. I used to go to the gym Monday through Friday, but now I go as much as possible because I am writing this book.

I have a bowl of sauerkraut or a bowl of yogurt for my snack. Sauerkraut is not my favorite, but I eat it for good health. Sometimes, I munch on my favorite nuts, celery, or cheeses. I was reading and watching information about how dairy is bad for us. I ignore that – I need nutrients from dairy for my hair, bones, and teeth.

Dairy has a lot of controversy around lactose intolerant, low-fat, and low sugar. If lactose intolerant, we must find something suitable for us that provides the same nutrients as dairy. We must be careful with those low-fat and low-sugar foods. I always read the labels. If there is an ingredient that I cannot pronounce, I know it is not good for me. Low-fat and low sugar are not always good for us because these companies always take out natural ingredients and replace them with chemicals that are bad for us. I still have all my teeth, my hair is strong, and my bones are fine because I eat cheese, yogurt, cottage cheese, and blue cheese to get the natural nutrients in dairy.

For my lunch, I eat a small portion of leftover dinner or a green salad. At dinner time, I eat what my husband cooks. If the dinner is healthy, then I eat normally. If it is not, I eat smaller portions. I also ensure I squeeze in my smoothie at the end of the day. In my smoothie, I put apple cider vinegar

(ACV), lemon, my favorite in-season fruit, celery, a sprinkle of pink Himalayan salt, dry rosemary leaves, and cinnamon. Before bed, I drink chamomile tea for a good night's rest.

I try to avoid white flour, white sugar, white rice, vegetable oil, hydrogenated oil, preservatives, additives, canned food, and processed food, but I am not too strict. Corn syrup is my biggest enemy. I avoid fast food and cut back on eating out at restaurants. However, restaurants are better than fast food because they offer more healthy choices. Occasionally, we have to go out with family and friends, which is okay – everything in moderation. More healthy diet tips, nutrition, and recipes are in Chapters XII, XIII, and XIV.

CHAPTER II:
Self-Care

When we hear "self-care," we often think of indulgent relaxation like taking a hot bath, spending a day at the spa, pouring a second glass of wine, or cutting an extra piece of the pie. While these habits have instant gratification effects, we must establish stable, repeatable, and sustainable self-care habits to live healthy lifestyles. Another form of self-care pertains to a long-term commitment to avoiding health complications.

What is self-care?

Self-care is taking care of ourselves through things we do regularly to support and promote our physical and mental health.   Individuals engage in some form of self-care every day from food choices and sleep to rest and exercise.

Self-care is also one of the first things to be put aside in times of stress, especially for those who are primary caregivers, including people caring for elderly relatives, parents of young children, healthcare providers, and first responders. These are people who often put the well-being of others above themselves. This is a big problem.

Three Fundamentals and Examples of Self-Care

There are many ways that we can exhibit self-care, but there are three main pillars to incorporate into our daily lives: physical well-being, emotional and mental well-being, and spiritual well-being.

Physical Well-being

Paying attention to our physical well-being means taking care of our physical bodies. Some examples of self-care for our physical well-being include:

- Eat healthy, well-balanced meals.
- Walk or exercise.
- Drink water
- Practice good hygiene
- Have a cup of tea.
- Take a relaxing shower or bath.
- Sit in the sunlight and try to get out of the house at least once daily.

Emotional and Mental Well-being

Emotional well-being relates to how we manage our thoughts, feelings, and emotions through all the ups, downs, celebrations, and obstacles that life throws our way. A person with balanced emotional health is aware of their mental state and emotions and has strategies to deal with both everyday situations and the up and down events that occur throughout their lives. Emotional and mental well-being is essential to our overall health and wellness. Some examples of emotional and mental self-care include:

- Take the time to understand our own feelings – we should monitor our feelings and behaviors for signs of distress, depression, or anxiety.
- Read a book.
- Listen to music or a podcast.
- Reflect on things we're grateful for
- Stay engaged in our social circles – call or text a friend, attend group gatherings, or visit with family (in person or online)
- Continue to do things that bring joy, such as hobbies, volunteering, working, or continued learning.

Spiritual Well-being

Spiritual well-being expands our sense of purpose and meaning in life, including our morals and ethics. It is essential to note this may or may not involve religious activities. It is different for everyone. Some examples of spiritual self-care include:

- Take time to pray, meditate or do meaningful spiritual practices.
- Speak to a religious leader to help make sense of current situations.
- Explore our own beliefs; this may or may not be affiliated with an organized religious group.
- Connect with nature.
- Engage in self-reflection.

We should not expect to incorporate all these things in our daily lives but remember to do something daily that helps us with our emotional, spiritual, and physical well-being. Remember, we cannot pour from an empty cup. We must first take care of and love ourselves.

Loving Ourselves

Loving ourselves is one of the most important things we can do to achieve a satisfying, meaningful, and joy-filled life. In a nutshell, loving ourselves is the ultimate form of self-care. Research studies related to wellness indicate that those who take good care of themselves and make healthy lifestyle choices are healthier, happier, more productive, miss less work, and have lower health costs. Here are some foundations to develop healthy habits for loving ourselves.

- **Make Ourselves THE Priority** – Many people fall into the trap of putting everyone else's needs first. They prioritize their children, spouse, friends, or dependent family members while never taking a moment out for themselves. This is not a realistic or healthy behavior because, if kept up, they'll soon drain their own tank. Once the tank is emptied, there is nothing more to give. That's why it is crucial to make ourselves our number one priority, not just a priority, but our number one priority. We must take time to recharge, take a breather, and put ourselves first. If we don't, it is a recipe for disaster. Just remember, to love others and be loved in return, we must first love ourselves.

- **Stop Criticizing Ourselves** – Each one of us, by virtue of being human, has some degree of insecurity. Perfection is not a good state. The reality is nobody is perfect, and nobody comes from a perfect family, yet many people judge themselves unmercifully for the slightest shortcomings. We criticize ourselves far more often and much more harshly than others judge us! We tell ourselves things like "being too ugly." If we tell ourselves these things too often, they become a reality. We must stop focusing on the negatives in every situation and instead find ways to see the positives. Whenever we have thoughts of criticism, shame, or guilt, we must find ways to turn those thoughts around.

- **Self-Praise** – One of the easiest ways to become more confident is to praise ourselves more often. Praise helps to build self-esteem and nurtures feelings of self-worth. Criticism, however, tears us down and can leave us feeling demoralized and hollow. When we belittle ourselves, we destroy hope which can have disastrous consequences. Learning how to become aware of and shift to a more positive and praise-filled internal dialogue is important. It may feel like confidence comes from outside sources, but our confidence completely relies on what we believe about ourselves. Now, this doesn't mean walking around pridefully boasting about every little thing; it means acknowledging our own capabilities, skills, and other positive qualities to encourage ourselves and expand our strengths.

Instead of focusing on the negatives in every situation, we should broaden our view and find the positives. What did we do well in a particular situation? Did we learn something from a challenging environment or interaction or discover a new way to do something?

Focusing on these positives, congratulating ourselves for what we did well, and noting the new knowledge we gained are positive ways to praise ourselves and build self-confidence.

- **Take Care of Our Bodies** – Many people turn to alcohol, drugs, smoking, and overeating to numb emotional pain or fight stress. Although these may work in the short term, over the long haul, these behaviors can often bring with them adverse outcomes which only serve to make our lives worse instead of better. We should respect and nurture our bodies by eating a healthy, well-balanced diet, exercising regularly, brushing our teeth, keeping ourselves clean and well-groomed, and getting enough sleep every night. Taking care of our bodies improves our health and mental outlook.

- **Be Our Own Best Friend** – We know ourselves better than anyone else, so it's in our best interest to love ourselves. There's one truth in life, and that is that we must go to bed each night and wake up each morning with ourselves. We know all our faults and all of our strengths. We know what makes us laugh and what makes us cry. So, who is better to be our best friend than ourselves? We must show ourselves the same compassion and empathy as a best friend or loved one. We should learn to enjoy our own company.

- **Stop Scaring Ourselves** – Many people let their negative thoughts spiral out of control. They obsess over terrifying worst-case scenarios and what-ifs. For example, if we have a stomach ache, thoughts immediately consider it might be cancer. Another scenario could be a co-worker or boss getting angry and snapping at us, and we automatically assume we will be fired. These thoughts can be terrifying, anxiety-provoking, and paralysing. These reactions can cause us to act inappropriately under the circumstances. It is okay to take a moment and breathe. Then replace these negative scenarios with a positive mental image. It can be a beautiful sunrise, a bouquet of flowers, the Bahamas, or anything that brings positive or calming feelings. Suppose we practice this whenever we find negative thoughts spiralling out of control. In that case, we will eventually succeed in keeping away the initial reaction to jump to worst-case scenarios and avoid unnecessary stress.

Self-Care Recommendations for Individuals with Diabetes

Diabetes can be the catalyst that contributes to long-term damage to the body and organs, including the eyes, kidneys, heart, nervous system, and blood vessels. Seven essential self-care behaviors predict good outcomes for people with diabetes: healthy eating, physical activity, monitoring blood sugar levels regularly, compliance with medication plans, good problem-solving skills, developing healthy coping skills, and applying risk-reduction behaviors.

For people with diabetes, or a family history of diabetes, it is recommended to adopt the following behaviors and self-care tactics:

- **Annual Eye Exam** – While seeing our optometrist regularly is part of maintaining good eye care. It is also recommended for adults with diabetes to see an ophthalmologist annually to get an annual dilated eye exam which can check for early signs of micro-vascular issues that commonly affect people with diabetes. The ophthalmologist can check the retina, at the back of the eye, for retinopathy – a condition characterized by blurred vision or partial blindness caused by damage to blood vessels in the eye. They can also check the macula at the retina's center for diabetic macular edema. Our annual eye exams are essential to the early detection and treatment of these conditions should they present themselves.

- **Caring For Feet** – We should always check the skin and webs of the toes for any open lesions or sores, which could be signs of the effects of diabetes on the body. We should also ensure that nails are trimmed straight to avoid ingrown toenails. Diabetes inhibits blood circulation, which could cause an ingrown toenail to quickly change from a painful but temporary nuisance to a life-changing issue. Additionally, wearing closed-toed shoes can help prevent foot injuries which diabetes effects on the body could also worsen.

- **Good Oral Hygiene** – Practicing good oral hygiene includes brushing teeth and flossing right after eating, minimizing the effects of gingivitis and periodontitis. If these diseases develop, they can contribute to blood glucose irregularity. Visiting a dentist twice a year can help catch early symptoms.

- **Checking the Skin** – A regular part of maintaining our bodies is inspecting the skin for discoloration or dryness. When skin is dry or discoloured, these factors can make the skin susceptible to scrapes and sores, especially when dehydrated. We should also note and discuss any uneven hair distribution or loss with our doctor, as this can signify more significant health issues like diabetes. Drinking water and staying hydrated keeps skin and hair strong and healthy.

- **Maintaining Sexual Health** – Even though this topic can be uncomfortable, it is still important to address. Many types of diabetes-related sexual dysfunction symptoms stem from blood vessel damage.

Blood vessel damage can also be the underlying cause of other major health issues affecting the heart, kidneys, eyes, and damage to the nervous system. Some symptoms to look for:

- o Increased urination, in both men and women, can often be a sign of diabetes or other more significant health issues.

- o For women, checking for recurring yeast infections or abnormal discharge is critical for detecting diabetes-related symptoms. Many women with diabetes often report sexual problems, which include loss of libido, issues with natural lubrication, arousal, and even pain. These can be signs of diabetes, but if not treated can also cause more significant problems, such as difficulty with pregnancy and depression.

- o In men with diabetes, sexual dysfunction often occurs in the form of erectile dysfunction and low libido. Erectile dysfunction often correlates with diabetes-related nerve damage typically caused by poorly controlled glucose levels. Poorly maintained sexual health in men can have larger impacts on overall health, such as emotional pain and the inability to maintain romantic relationships.

- **Reduce Stress** – When enduring physical and emotional stress, it can make it difficult to follow a treatment plan. This difficulty in aligning and following an individualized plan can leave people feeling hopeless or unmotivated. Stress manifests differently for every person, so stress reduction will also be very different for every person, but it is important to do our best to reduce stress. We should discuss methods with loved ones or caregivers and keep track of what has worked and what has not.

- **Reporting Symptoms & Utilizing Support Systems** – We should consult with our doctors regularly on any symptoms out of the ordinary, especially numbness or tingling. Numbness can be a sign of nerve damage, called peripheral neuropathy, the most common type of neuropathy associated with diabetes. This condition typically affects the feet and legs first, followed by the hands and arms. The symptoms of peripheral neuropathy are often worse at night. They can include numbness, sharp pains or cramps, tingling or burning feeling, and reduced ability to feel pain or temperature changes. This is especially dangerous for older patients who have lost the sense in their limbs and cannot test if the bath water is too hot or feel for open wounds that could get infected without proper care and treatment.

When we think of "self-care," it often implies solitude. However, it's recommended that people talk about routines, struggles, and wins with family members, caregivers, or friends. Additionally, it is a powerful tool to seek out support groups in your local community or online to find support and others going through a similar situation to discuss what we're experiencing. It's hard to stay motivated and on track when we are alone and do not feel supported, but it is up to us to share or seek the support we need to succeed.

Why is self-care important?

Those who take good care of themselves and make healthy lifestyle choices are generally healthier, happier, more productive, miss less work, and have lower healthcare-related costs. It is essential to take good care of ourselves and our well-being first in order for us to take good care of others. It is just like when on an airplane, the flight attendant gives the safety instructions, and they always reiterate that if any passengers are traveling with young children or those who need assistance, to put their own oxygen mask on first. Then they can assist children and others who need help.

We often neglect our physical, social, spiritual, and emotional health. This may happen due to lack of time, inability to step away from responsibilities, fatigue, or guilt for enjoying ourselves. Ignoring our needs invariably leads to chronic stress, burnout, and chronic inflammation. All of this can lead to long-term health problems, isolation, and disruption in usual relationships.

My research and reflection for this chapter were surprising to me. I thought all these years that I loved myself. Little did I know I loved others more than myself. Like the verse said:

30 And you shall love the LORD your God with all your heart, with all your soul, with all your mind, and with all your strength. This is the first commandment. 31And the second like it, is this, 'You shall love your neighbor as yourself.' - Mark 12:30-31 (NKJV)

I am willing to learn and grow. Now I know I must love, trust, honor, respect, and appreciate myself before I can love others. I must make myself my priority and allow myself to make mistakes. I trust myself to make good decisions for myself. I have to stop waiting for the right time to do the things I want to do. If I wait, it might never come. If I want to do something or try something, I am doing it now. Counting my blessings makes me feel good all the time. I am always thankful for life, good health, friends, and family. It doesn't matter what happens to me in the future. I know it is going to be great and wonderful.

CHAPTER III:
Belief

The meaning of "believe" is to accept (something) as true, genuine, or real. It also can be defined as having a wholehearted conviction, opinion, or thought. Novelist Franz Kafka once said, "By believing passionately in something that still does not exist, we create it. The nonexistent is whatever we have not sufficiently desired." In the Bible, Hebrews 11:1 (NKJV) says, "Now faith is the substance of things hoped for, the evidence of things not seen."

Just believing is not a guarantee of success, but it is vital that we maintain confidence within ourselves that we will overcome any obstacles placed in our way. If we allow doubt to take over, we will subconsciously damage or obstruct our own efforts and success.

The Law of Attraction, for example, states whatever we focus our energy on will come to us. By focusing on what we want to achieve, the law of attraction says we emit positive energy to attract those desires and achievements our way. The unconscious attraction is one of the strongest forces acting upon us - pulling us to be who we believe we are - so we must always have positive beliefs.

Benefits of Believing

There are a plethora of reasons why having a strong belief set and belief system are important, but there are five benefits to believing and why it is especially important.

- **Create the Right Mindset and Inspire Yourself to Act** -- When we believe we can achieve something or attract something to our lives, it sets the foundation for strong and constructive action toward our goals. We must create a mindset that will give us motivation, discipline, and mental capacity to carry us through to the completion of our goals and desires. Once we have established this foundation, we can actually see ourselves accomplishing something and arriving at the desired finish line. Then we are highly motivated to work toward the goals we have set out for ourselves. Then, we will continue working on this until we finally get to the finish line.

- **Spot Opportunities and Trust the Process** – When we have a strong belief set, our subconscious mind becomes a goal-seeking machine and will constantly look for things to reaffirm our positive and negative self-beliefs. Our unconscious mind does not care about our goals, desires, or ambitions. However, it does look for opportunities to highlight information it can find to validate and support our internal beliefs. Research suggests that it is possible, through conditioning, to retrain our unconscious minds to seek information to reaffirm positive thoughts and help us spot new opportunities to help us achieve our goals, even those we may have overlooked.

While we can retrain our subconscious to spot opportunities, we must also remember to trust the process. Failure and unsuccessful attempts are part of the process and likely temporary setbacks. When we experience constant failure, we can't give up. The next attempt may be the pivotal moment for success.

- **Increases Self-Confidence** – Belief that a difficult task is possible ultimately gives us the confidence to complete the task at hand. Believing in something strengthens the neurons in our brains and increases our belief in the ultimate desired outcome. We then start to feed our brains with positive thinking and self-belief affirmations. We start leaving little to no space for negative thoughts; even when they come from time to time, our confidence beats them quickly. The more belief we have in accomplishing tasks toward our desired outcome ultimately increases our self-confidence. Our confidence grows not only for the tasks at hand and the desired result but for ourselves, our strengths, and capabilities…and honestly, if you don't believe in yourself to succeed, then why would anybody else?

- **Create Belief in Others** – We must accept that despite our efforts and achievements along the way, there is no such thing as a completely self-made person. We've all had support, guidance, and direction at some stage in our lives. From support and direction as a child to financial support from parents or a financial institution. It could be mentorship from a colleague or community member. These and many more have all played a part in our current success. When we develop and display a level of confidence that demonstrates to those around us our belief and determination, quite often, this will be the "communication" it takes that inspires them to either take a chance on us or support us on our journey to our goals.

- **Reduce Stress and Have Peace of Mind** – Building our self-confidence and belief in our abilities to achieve existing goals and new challenges can significantly reduce stress and give us peace of mind in both our personal and professional lives. As confidence grows, areas in our lives such as personal conflict, tight deadlines, or public speaking will no longer take a toll on our mental resources. This allows us more cognitive energy to take on new challenges. On the other hand, when we feed our stress hormones, this not only has a detrimental effect on our peace of mind but can also affect our creative process and physical well-being. That said, we must build self-confidence by believing in ourselves, reducing stress, and increasing our peace of mind. These factors will boost mental wellness and physical well-being.

Believe In Yourself

Believing in yourself means having confidence in your goals, desires, and abilities to reach your desired outcomes. It means trusting yourself to do what you need to and that those efforts will result in the desired outcomes. Several factors and psychological experiences contribute to our belief in ourselves. Those include a mixture of critical psychological experiences like self-worth, self-confidence, self-trust, self-respect, and autonomy. While there are many ways to develop and nurture belief in yourself, here are five powerful steps to overcome any obstacles in the way of developing confidence and belief in yourself.

- **Nurture your Strengths** – When struggling with confidence, we tend to focus on the negatives or things we can't do. Our human nature is to focus on these weaknesses because we feel failure and weakness much differently and more keenly than success and achievement. We also find ourselves trying to work on and fix our flaws. Instead, we should determine and identify our strengths to build these up and get the most mileage out of them. To build up confidence right away, stop beating weaknesses with a stick, but instead, discover what you're already good at, and work at becoming even greater at those strengths.

- **Be Your Own Coach** – Even though we may be good at something, if we don't believe in ourselves, we won't believe when others cheer us on or express how proud they are of us. That's why the greatest coaches don't just cheerlead from the sideline but instead find success in identifying strengths and developing talent. So how can you be your own coach? Identify the parts of your life that you are satisfied with and keep an eye on where you ultimately want to be. Seek out tools and knowledge to help develop your talents and strengths. Then, take action. Set one big goal at a time and break it down into smaller parts. Success in each small part, no matter how small or insignificant it may seem, adds up to visible progress.

- **Embrace Who You Are** – When we embrace who we are and what is important to us, we build self-confidence. You must understand what makes you unique and celebrate those things. Embracing yourself is best accomplished in baby steps. A good starting point is to write down what is important to you. Do this several times and over time. Each time you'll get closer to identifying and uncovering the core values that make you who you are.

Are you a people pleaser? Although being nice or keeping the peace may seem like the way to go, after so many years, I felt terrible. I am sure some people will not like the new me, but I've learned to be okay with that. I am not doing it to them or for them; I'm doing it for myself. I talk to myself a lot. I remind myself that this is my journey, not theirs. I believe change is possible. It is the way to grow. I say this to remind myself that it is okay to step away from the expectations of others and do new things often. We can learn so much from ourselves when we step out of routine and just doing what is comfortable. We should mix things up and do new things often. You'll be impressed by what you learn about yourself along the way! I know I have been!

- **Be Uncomfortable** – To really make a change in life, we have to step out of our comfort zone and do things differently. Do weird things. Do things that make us super uncomfortable, experiment with who we are, and try things we haven't tried before. If we want a different path in life, we must do it ourselves. Blaze our own trail through experimenting and acting on our ideas. Our capabilities and potential will be reflected back. The good news is that when we start to do more new things, the fear becomes fun. There are still challenges, though, we may have to go through real anxiety and work on ways to manage it, but the results will be worth it. Self-improvement can be scary, but those who have gone through it will tell you it is worth it.

- **Believe You Can Succeed, and You Will** – Belief is the most powerful thing to have, and we can completely change our lives by changing our beliefs. In life, we can either see possibilities ahead or dwell on the obstacles in front of us. Which will you choose?

A fixed mindset is a limited thinking pattern in which we tell ourselves that we are *stuck* with the skills and capabilities we have right now. This mindset can be detrimental to our success. Instead, we should adopt a growth mindset, where we start believing that we can change and improve. Start investing time and effort in becoming that "someone" we want to be. Nothing is stopping us. No matter what our dreams are, once we wholeheartedly believe that it will come true, that's when the adventure begins. Always think of success and have the courage to believe big. Do not allow thoughts of failure to conquer your mind. When we believe in ourselves and what we do, we are better than what our mind tells us.

Believe and Achieve Your Dreams

When we have established a clear and precise picture of who we are, who we want to be, and what we want to do or have, and then developed our belief and confidence in that dream, we must achieve it. Some believe achievement can be broken down into simple steps. Others believe it is not that clean or easy. For those who achieve great things, there are seven steps in the process that can be repeatable. Once we start to develop and apply these habits, we'll be well on our way to achieving our dreams.

- **Dream It --** Start with a vision. Everything starts in the heart and mind. Every great achievement begins with someone's vision. They dared to dream and believe it was possible. They identified the things it would take to achieve the desired outcome. Many people go through life without identifying their vision, objectives, or desires. Without this, they live life reacting to the world around them and simply follow the crowd rather than living a purposeful and driven life.

  Take time to ask yourself, "What if?" or "What does success mean to me and look like in my life?" What lifestyle would you want to live if you had all the resources available? It's okay to think and dream big. Don't let negative thoughts or temporary past failures discourage you. In this situation, you want to be a "dreamer." Dream of the possibilities for yourself, your family, and others. If you've ever had a dream that you let grow cold, re-ignite that dream! It's time to add fuel to the fire and fan the flames. Life is too short to give up or live life within the boundaries of our comfort zones and routines.

- **Believe It –** Believe in your dreams. When you start believing, that's when the true adventure begins. Your dreams should be big. They should be something that is seemingly just outside of grasp and current capabilities, but they must still be believable. You must be able to realistically say that this dream or goal is achievable if certain things happen. If you work hard enough and put in the effort to learn something new or accept the help of others, it can be done. I like to think an excellent example of this is myself, at 72 years old, who has never been a writer and does not have any training in literature, has been able to learn how to write a book and, with some help, also self-publish it! A big but believable and achievable dream. A bad example is someone who is unhealthy and has not trained physically to dream that he can wake up tomorrow and run a marathon. However, if he gave himself several months to train and put in the effort, he could dream of running a marathon in the future.

- **Envision It** – Some of the greatest achievers have a habit of envisioning what they want or need to accomplish. Once they've established their desired goal or outcome, they picture themselves achieving it, and reaping the rewards, before it has even happened. You may still be sitting on a folding chair in your garage but can envision walking around the c-suite offices at the corporate headquarters of your multi-million-dollar company. The greatest athletes imagine their next game-winning play before they even make the shot. Training our brains to think this way controls our bodies to carry out the dream.

- **Talk About It** – One of the main reasons that many dreams never go anywhere is that no one is talking about them. If we keep our dreams to ourselves, it becomes a dream that only lives inside our own mind. If we want to accomplish our goals, we need to talk about them. The more people we talk about our dreams with, the more support and help we have to achieve our dreams. Also, the more we say it aloud, the more we believe in ourselves and our abilities to accomplish our vision. If we are talking about it, then it must be possible, right?

- **Plan It** – Sound familiar? We already talked about how important a plan is for overall healthy living, but it's also essential to have a plan to accomplish our dreams. Every dream must take the form of a plan. The old saying, "You get what you wish for," is untrue. Dreams won't just happen overnight or on their own. We need to sit down regularly and plan out our strategy for achieving the goals we've set for ourselves. Unless we have a plan and a process to work toward, then we have nothing to work on and no small steps to take in order to get to our desired outcomes.

- **Work It** – Boy, wouldn't life be great if we could just quit before this step!? Unfortunately, that's not the case. The ones who are most successful are usually the hardest workers. They are working hard while the rest of the world sits on their sofas and watches reruns. The best equation for achieving our goals and dreams is to work on short-term tasks multiplied by time equals long-term success. In other words, if we follow our plan and work on each short-term task, these add up to the success of our long-term, bigger-picture dream over time.

- **Enjoy It** – Celebrating when we have reached our goals is essential. When we have accomplished our dream, we must be sure to enjoy it. We should plan to reward ourselves for milestones along the way. We should also plan for a larger reward when we have reached the desired outcome and living out the dream. We should also help others enjoy our success. We should be gracious and generous and use our success to better others. We should use our success to encourage others to dream big and achieve their goals. Once we've achieved our dream, it is time to go back to number 1, but this time our objective should be a little bit bigger. Dream, believe, achieve, repeat!

So, what happens if our dreams don't come true exactly as we've planned? Not to worry, it's okay. If things don't go according to plan, I believe it's because our Lord has other plans. Earlier this year, I thought of volunteering because I felt like giving back some of my blessings to our community. I asked myself what can I do? Working with children came to mind. I enjoyed working with K-12 in the past, and I saw the opportunity and jumped on it! Then, I found that the application process was so hard. I felt like I was applying for a real job. Wait a minute! I just wanted to volunteer my precious time - nothing comes out of it if it's more trouble than it is worth. Little did I know God had other plans for my time.

We'll never know why some things don't go as we planned. Maybe God was stopping me from being around children so I wouldn't risk getting sick with Covid-19. A child might get injured during my time with them, and I'll get sued. I am healthy, active, and vibrant, but I'm still 72. Who knows? Now, I am spending my free time writing, reading, and sharing my experience and knowledge - in a much more meaningful way through writing, which I enjoy.

What I Believe

I believe everything that has been happening to me is from God. All my blessings come from HIM. When I go through tough times, I know HE is telling me I am not going in the right direction. I must change what I am doing.

"Jesus said to him, 'If you can believe, all things are possible to him who believes.'" - Mark 9:23 (NKJV)

Whatever I want in life, I believe I can make it happen. Some people believe in their ability to make it happen, and some don't. The truth is, they're both right. It's up to us to believe one way or the other and to make it happen. We're responsible for all the blessings that come our way to enjoy. If we want something, we'll find a way. If we don't, we'll find excuses not to. Sure, you have heard that before. You don't get what you pray for; you don't get what you wish for. You get what you believe in and work for. People have even been healed because they chose to believe in (and work toward) better health.

Watching how my life gets better as time goes by, started from my thoughts. It creates my life. I am aware of what I am thinking as much as possible. Life gives me something to do. I believe, at this time; it is to write so that I can share my learning and experiences with others. There are thoughts that I need to let go of because it doesn't serve me anymore. There are good thoughts that will improve my life, and I am looking forward to them.

Everybody has their belief system. Some might be true for them, but not for me. My life has improved since last year, when I changed some of my beliefs and mindset. Now, I appreciate my life, and it is always good. Somehow, by changing how I think, I have more appreciation and joy in my life. It is the same life, but I am being mindful and paying attention to my thoughts, what brings me joy and blessings, and what I now enjoy. I can't express how happy I am with my newfound happiness. It truly is amazing!

I had a situation recently, where a family member told me how to do something. I nodded in agreement, but I was telling myself that might be good for you but not for me. However, I did not say it out loud. She has her path, and I have mine. I am happy with my path. I can make decisions for myself. It has been a good year, and I believe it will be better years ahead. With each challenge in life that I can overcome, I become more intelligent and experienced. I have become very smart and now make better choices and decisions for myself. My thoughts are powerful. I make sure my thoughts are helping me progress and produce. If my thoughts hurt me or others in some way, then I reject that thought as fast as I can. I go back to my beautiful views and am happier with my choices and decisions because of my positive thoughts. God is good, and life is wonderful. It is a miracle.

CHAPTER IV:
Identifying Positivity & Negativity

Positive Attitude

Having a positive attitude means being optimistic about the situation at hand, current interaction, and yourself. It means approaching unpleasant situations with more positivity and productivity. People with positive attitudes remain hopeful and see the best in everything, even in difficult situations. In contrast, those with negative mindsets may be more pessimistic and disagreeable and typically expect the worst outcomes.

It is important to have a positive attitude because it can help equip us with the tools and ability to cope with stress in better ways. With a positive mental attitude, our language becomes more optimistic, consequently impacting our habits, values, and future. We are also often able to deal with stress and negative situations in a much healthier way. When we adopt a positive attitude, we naturally become more optimistic. Rather than thinking, "the grass is greener on the other side," we start to feel and believe we're already on the greener side. We begin to feel and adapt differently to disappointments and setbacks. When this happens we bounce back more quickly. Don't get me wrong, they'll still be challenging, but we'll be able to cope and bounce back much quicker. When unfavorable situations occur, we will be able to accept that things turned out the way they did rather than being in denial.

We also become more empathetic and understanding toward others when we have a positive attitude. We learn to see the thoughts behind people's actions and why they may have acted the way they did rather than jumping to a harmful conclusion. This also helps us become more grateful. With a positive outlook, we are thankful for the good things in work and life. We start to approach every day with an appreciative mind and outlook.

Building a positive mindset starts with self-talk and introspection and is based on a detailed analysis of the world around you. We can change the trajectory of our lives by achieving a positive mindset. Having a positive mindset is a game changer, as it will further elevate and improve our attitude and behaviors and make us happier people in the process.

Creative Ways to Keep a Positive Attitude

You may be asking, "Okay, Cora, if it's so great, how do we create and keep a positive attitude?" Great Question! There are many ways to help shift our mindset to a more positive outlook. Here are some ideas and habits that I have adapted to help create and maintain my positive attitude. Give some of these a try and see what works for you.

- **Start a Gratitude Journal** – A gratitude journal is a diary in which someone keeps a record of things they are grateful for. Keeping a gratitude journal is a popular tool and practice in positive psychology. There is no right or wrong way to keep a gratitude journal, but here are some ideas to get you started. Write down things you are grateful for, try and start with 3 to 5 items. (Hint: Don't just do this in your head, actually write it down.) The things you write down may seem unimportant, and some may be significant milestones. Write it all down. The goal of this exercise is to remember good experiences and things in life and the good emotions that come with that event or occasion.

  There are many ways to maintain a gratitude journal. Some start by purchasing a guided journal with daily and monthly prompts. Others keep a notebook where they write things down regularly. There are even a lot of free prompts to be found online. Whichever route you choose, remember to utilize your gratitude journal regularly.

- **Always have something to look forward to and enjoy every day** – Even though we may be tired after work or feel overwhelmed with our already packed schedules, we must craft our days and routines to include more than work or obligations. We must learn to regularly pencil in some fun time and relaxation or self-spoil time. We should always have something to look forward to. We should also ensure that we plan to do at least one thing every day that we enjoy – this way, we can ensure that we at least attempt to enjoy every day. The point is, we must find healthy ways to balance work and personal life. We must also balance what we do for others with what we do for ourselves.

- **Include More Humor in Your Day** – Humor and laughter genuinely are some of the best medicine out there! Laughter can increase endorphins, release tension in our bodies, and helps to relieve stress. These are significant short-term effects on our mindsets and bodies. There are also great long-term benefits of including laughter as part of our day regularly. The positive thoughts and vibes we receive with laughter can release neuropeptides that fight stress and help us cope with difficult situations. When we include more jokes and humor into our daily lives, we can also use humor to lighten and cope easier with difficult situations - thus avoiding unnecessary stress on our bodies and minds.

- **Practice Meditation** – Meditation can help us to decrease stress and anxiety, and in the long run, help improve mental and spiritual health. Even 5 - 10 minutes of meditation daily is a great way to improve mental stability and routine. If you're unfamiliar with meditation, start with deep breathing and clearing your mind. Simple methods like this are a great starting point and take little effort to help find balance.

- **Listen to Music that Matches Your Mood and Environment** – When we are happy, we can enhance our mood with happy and upbeat tunes. There have even been recent studies that indicate certain sounds and tones can help boost productivity, whether at work or home.

  It is also okay to listen to sad music when we are sad. Psychology professors have studied the effects sad music can have on our moods. The conclusion was that many people use sad songs as a form of mood enhancement, as many consider sad music to be "beautiful" and full of expression. This helps people start to feel better about their current environment or circumstances and can distract them from dwelling on negative thoughts and situations.

- **Focus on the Long-term** – We can often avoid unnecessary stress when we take a moment to step back and look at the long-term implications of a negative or stressful situation that is in front of us at a given moment. If we can focus on the long-term, we can evaluate if we react or engage in conflict, will the outcomes be beneficial long-term? If not, it may be better for us to find empathy and look for the root of the problem in the current moment. It may be that the person we are interacting with is just having a bad day or a negative interaction with someone else. Positive thinking will encourage the other person to feel better about the situation and themselves.

The Impacts of a Positive Attitude

Positive thinking arms us with better approaches to reality and can help improve four essential areas in our lives:

- **Physical Health** – When we're under a lot of stress or often feel angry or anxious, the organ that suffers the most is our heart. Studies have found that people with a positive attitude typically have healthier habits, including eating healthier foods and exercising more regularly. They often drink less alcohol and rarely smoke compared to those with a less positive mindset. In general, people with a positive attitude experience less stress and can focus on information that helps strengthen their mood and immune system. Ultimately, those with a positive attitude have been found to have a longer lifespan!

- **Mental Health** – When we allow a negative attitude or outlook to take over, we experience excessive worrying, typical for people under stress. Positive thinking helps us grow mentally and emotionally. We look forward to a healthy future ahead of us.

- **Relationships** – It is no secret that optimistic people are simply more pleasant to be around. We don't need science to tell us that we'd rather spend time with someone who smiles, listens, has an empathetic approach, and sees the good even in bad situations. When we have a negative mindset, it affects all the relationships in our lives, including family, friends, romantic and professional – therefore affecting all aspects of our lives. When we adopt and maintain a positive attitude, people are more likely to want to spend quality time with us, allowing us to nurture all those relationships in all aspects of our lives.

- **Career** – Psychologist Sonya Lyubomirsky and her colleagues discovered that happier employees are generally more productive. They are also more creative and receive better evaluations from their supervisors. As a result, they also make more money! This means that both employees and the organization benefit from instilling a positive mindset. We must work cooperatively with our work organizations to create, engage, and maintain a positive culture and work environment in our workplaces for ourselves, our colleagues, and our organizations. This means that we become happier, healthier, more connected, and ultimately wealthier.

Negativity Bias and Forms of Negativity

Negativity occurs when someone has a worrisome or gloomy outlook on life. This can and does happen to anyone and everyone at some point in life. However, persistent negative thoughts can link to a person's mental and physical health as well as social well-being. Negativity is typically temporary, specifically when a person experiences an adverse event or period of difficulty.

Negativity bias is the natural tendency for people to acknowledge negative triggers more readily and mull over these events with more detail and attention. When we enter this positive-negative asymmetry, it is referred to as negativity bias. In negativity bias, people feel and connect more with the sting of failure or struggle more strongly than they accept and enjoy the feelings of praise and positivity. Pessimistic people often develop a negative mindset as a form of self-preservation in response to an adverse or difficult situation. It is most often a product of insecurity and depression but can showcase a variety of traits and reactions. Long-term negativity can often manifest as cynicism, a general distrust of people and their motives, and hostility, which causes people to be generally unfriendly towards others. There is also filtering when people only notice the bad in what should be a happy experience or memory. There is polarizing thinking; people think if something or someone is not perfect, they must be horrible.

Psychologist Aaron T. Beck initially theorized cognitive distortion in the 1960s. Essentially, cognitive distortion is when our mind distorts what we see and attach to our experiences.

There are various forms of cognitive distortion, but the most common and identifiable include:

- **All-or-nothing thinking** – When people view themselves/their experiences as only complete success or failure.

- **Jumping to conclusions** – We do this all the time. Instead of letting the facts and evidence bring us to a logical conclusion and reality, we set our sights on an assumed outcome (often negative). When doing this, we seek evidence to back up our decision, often ignoring the evidence of the contrary. We often assume what others think or plan, usually a negative assumption of how things will turn out.

- **Catastrophizing** – When someone is always assuming and expecting the worst possible outcome. This leads to a lot of stress and reactive behaviour instead of proactive decision-making.

- **Identifying** – When people overgeneralize past experiences and those outcomes to all future similar experiences.

- **Labelling and Personalization** – This is when we label ourselves in a negative way - it ultimately affects how we feel about ourselves. If we label ourselves bad at something, we will always feel negative when doing that activity. Additionally, personalization is when we take things personally and take on "blame" even when we don't have control over the situation or the outcome.

- **Emotional reasoning** – This can be like jumping to conclusions as it also involves ignoring facts when drawing conclusions. Emotional reasoning occurs when we consider our feelings and emotions as evidence rather than objectively looking at facts. For example, if you are walking into a new place and feeling nervous, you may start to feel like you are in danger - even when there are no signs of danger.

Once we start identifying our negative thoughts and self-talk, we can replace the negative ones. We should challenge our negative thinking and explore more practical and realistic alternatives.

Ways to Avoid Negativity

We will inevitably experience things throughout life that will cause us negative thoughts. The negative mindset usually improves once matters are resolved, but negativity can also take root in us if we let it. So how do we avoid negativity? It's not always easy, but here are some ways to help identify our negative behavior and habits to help us process in a healthy way to get back to positivity.

- **Practice Mindfulness and Self-Awareness –** Mindfulness has its roots in meditation. It is the practice of detaching yourself from your thoughts and emotions and viewing them as an outside observer. Practicing mindfulness can help us become more conscious of our thoughts and build greater self-awareness. When we practice mindfulness, we can achieve self-awareness. That is, we become aware of how our thoughts impact our emotions and behaviours. The objective of mindfulness is to gain control of our emotional reactions to situations by allowing the thinking part of our brains to take over.

  Practicing mindfulness helps me become more conscious of my thoughts and build greater awareness of how it impacts my emotions and behaviour. Mindfulness helps me control my emotional reaction to situations and to allow my thinking brain to take over. I don't see the world now as a problem. I see the world as a challenge.

- **Notice Your Breath –** Mindfulness can weaken the chain of association that keeps you obsessing about and even wallowing in a setback. Mindfulness of breathing is an excellent place to start. It is easy to focus on our breath during daily activities and provides a clear anchor or support for mindfulness. The basic idea is to sit in a chair, relaxed but sitting up straight, and focus on your breathing. When you do this, notice the sensation it triggers throughout your body. Focus as the abdomen moves in and out and the air passes the tip of your nose. The breathing exercise feels comfortable and at ease. Mindful meditation should not be judgmental.

- **Cultivate Compassion –** Practice simple compassion. Focus on relieving suffering for others, which can help to feel less negative and may bring positive experiences or a sense of spontaneous joy. Compliment others regularly - keep an eye out for opportunities to applaud someone for a job well done at work or compliment a neighbor's beautiful garden. Hint: Make it even more meaningful by looking directly into the eyes of the person you are complimenting.

- **Express Gratitude Regularly** – Pay attention to the times you say, "thank you." When you do, look directly into the eyes of the person you are thanking and muster as much genuine gratitude as you can. Gratitude can inspire positive thoughts by helping focus on the good aspects of any event.

- **Notice the Good and Practice Saying Positive Things** – Start seeking out and recognizing the good things that bring joy and excitement. Look for the good characteristics you like and appreciate in yourself and those in people you regularly interact with. Write down one positive characteristic of yourself and one trait of someone you regularly interact with. Do this three times a day. Ideally, write down different characteristics each time, but if unsure or stuck, that's okay too. Keeping track of and acknowledging the good things about professional and personal lives will likely help maintain a positive mood.

- **Avoid Negative People and Negative Situations** – Both positivity and negativity can be contagious. If we keep as much distance from negative people, it can help influence our moods. On that same token, we should attempt to stay near positive people as their positivity will likely be contagious and help boost our mood.

- **Work with Negative Emotions and Bounce Back from Challenges** – Decrease negative emotions by trying a variant of "exposure therapy." Exposure therapy consists of progressively more direct exposure to cues that produce negative emotions which helps development of learning and healthy ways to relax. When experiencing negative feelings or thoughts, try rearranging your environment to promote a speedy recovery from adversity. Leave the situation where a setback occurred. Additionally, learn to live more in the moment. Avoid dwelling on past mistakes or being too worried about future events. These habits can affect current positivity and cause unnecessary stress.

The Effects of Negativity

We must be aware of the effects of prolonged negativity, which affects much more than just emotional health. Doctors have found people with pessimism and high negativity levels are more likely to suffer from cardiovascular and digestive issues and prolonged body aches and pains. Typically, they recover from sickness much slower than those with a positive mindset.

Studies have shown that a negative mindset and overall negativity can be linked to chronic headaches, chest pain, and fatigue. Additionally, people with a pessimistic outlook generally suffer from sleep problems, anxiety and depression, and even social withdrawal. There has been links between eating disorders and drastic changes in metabolism. These are signals that prolonged negativity can affect our overall well-being and may be the catalysts in our bodies for other health issues like diabetes or heart attack.

How Negativity and Positivity Impact My Life

It is no secret that optimistic people are simply more pleasant to be around. We don't need science to tell us that we would rather spend time with someone who smiles, listens, has an empathetic approach, and sees the good even in a bad situation.

I see how unhappy negative people are, and I'll do everything in my power not to be one. Negativity can ruin relationships and friendships. Those people I thought were unhappy must be full of negativity. They always seem to have a problem for every solution. They gossip a lot and are angry about nonsense. I can feel their doubts, and they drain me physically and mentally. I feel terrible when I am around them, which makes me not want to be around them. I learned that being around negativity affects me, and I realized I could not spend time with negative people and expect a beautiful life. Whatever I allow in my life becomes my life. Negative thoughts are my biggest enemy. I don't want to waste time on it if I can help it. It ruins my day. I choose to be happy. I want to keep seeing the good in people. Everybody has something good about them. I am going to learn what they are. I always try to be a positive influence, but if they influence me with their negativity, then I don't have a choice but to stay away from them. Happiness is a choice.

Changing my thoughts and behavior predicts my future. By becoming aware of my conscious mind, I am successful at removing all of the unnecessary and negative thoughts that linger in my head. Awareness creates energy in me. When I connect with my conscious mind, I realize my joy comes from within…not from my closet, the store, or another person.

I always choose to be pleasant and positive. What I think decides my day. When I wake up miserable, I attract more misery. My day is better, even with challenges, when I wake up with thankfulness and gratitude. Healthy living is more than exercise and eating right. It affects our whole life. Our choices, thoughts, actions, beliefs, and what we say and do make a difference. When we are happy and healthy, we are more likely to make better decisions and choices.

CHAPTER V:
Physical Health

The Role of Movement and Exercise

A healthy lifestyle for our bodies requires regular physical activity and hearty but balanced eating. Getting physical activity doesn't have to be an hour-plus-long trip to the gym. Just get up and move around throughout the day. Any form of moving our bodies is beneficial to our bodies. Try incorporating, into your daily routine, physical activities like gardening, housework, playing with pets and friends, or taking a walk. We are not meant to be trees. A sedentary lifestyle causes a lot of harm to the body. Those who are inactive are more likely to experience health complications like obesity, pain caused by muscles, and bones losing their strength. Inactive people also often have diabetes from a reduced metabolism which causes difficulty breaking down sugars and fats, or general illness from a weakened immune system.

Our bodies also need regular exercise, vital to our physical well-being and healthy bodies. Exercising regularly helps foster both brain and body wellness. Research studies have suggested that the top benefits of exercise include the following:

- **Improve Brain Health** – When we exercise regularly, we improve brain health which ultimately keeps us in a better mood and helps us to avoid depression and anxiety. Regular exercise is also linked with improved memory.

- **Weight Loss, Reduce Pain, and Overall Physical Health** – Studies have shown that inactivity is a significant factor in weight gain and obesity. Daily physical activity is recommended to reduce belly fat and decrease the development of chronic diseases. Regular exercise is crucial to healthy metabolism and can help reduce high blood pressure and cholesterol. When we exercise regularly, our bodies become stronger by building and maintaining muscle and bone strength. This, in turn, helps our bodies prevent chronic pain in muscles and joints. Regular exercise can strengthen the heart, improve blood circulation, tone muscles, and much more for our bodies!

- **Improved Energy Levels** – Exercise can be a natural energy boost for many people, including those with various medical conditions.

- **Skin Health** – Regular exercise can stimulate blood flow and induce skin adaptations that can help delay the appearance of aging.

- **Sleep and Relaxation Quality** – When we exercise, we sweat, which helps get rid of the toxins in our bodies. As our bodies flush those toxins and process stress and emotions, the result may be an improvement in sleep patterns and quality. Additionally, when our bodies are not holding on to as much stress, it allows us to relax and decompress.

- **Promote a Better Sex Life –** It has been proven that exercise boosts endorphins and hormones that can increase sex drive – which is essential for our relationship and sexual satisfaction. There are other health benefits to a healthy sex drive, including lower blood pressure and improved immune systems (did you know that sexual health experts have found sexually active people generally take fewer sick days?). Additionally, for women, it can help with improved bladder control.

Getting started is often the most challenging part, but once we get moving, it gets easier. When I interviewed Kathleen, she said, "before you pick up the phone, stretch and start walking. While talking on the phone, you will be distracted and not notice how many steps you are doing." I like this advice! I know many people don't want to go outside, let alone go walking, but try this idea next time you plan to call someone – and fill both your physical activity and social well-being meters at the same time! It is recommended that walking for just 30 minutes each day reduces the risks and effects of stroke and heart disease as well as helps manage the symptoms of high cholesterol and diabetes. Walking is mostly safe for all ages and an excellent place to start but find something that you find enjoyable and makes you happy. If you enjoy what you are doing, you're more likely to keep doing it, which will keep you moving!

If walking isn't your thing, that's okay. People of all ages are meant to be appropriately active. It's also important to keep in mind that exercise is typically categorized into three intensity levels: low, moderate, and vigorous. Physical activity does not always have to be vigorous to be beneficial. That said, we should incorporate light, low-level, and higher-intensity activities appropriate for our capabilities and lifestyle.

Aerobic exercise provides cardiovascular conditioning, which means that breathing controls the amount of oxygen that can make it to the muscles to help burn fuel and move. Some lower-impact forms of aerobic exercise include swimming, cycling, and walking. Some higher-impact forms include jogging, running, and jumping rope. You could also check for group classes like Zumba, Pilates, or Yoga at your local gym or community center.

We know that physical exercise is part of a healthy lifestyle, but what are the health benefits of regular movement? Obviously long term, activity helps to keep our bodies in shape, but regular exercise has some immediate benefits, like releasing endorphins which help relieve stress, and physical movement also helps emotions move through our bodies. Additionally, incorporating movement through other activities allows us to take a break from everyday challenges and responsibilities.

The bottom line is exercise offers incredible benefits that can improve nearly all aspects of our health. Adding movement and exercise to our routines can increase the production of hormones that make us feel happier, improve mood and confidence, help us sleep better, and improve the overall health of our bodies. Just start a little, the next day a little more. Before you know it, you are doing a lot more. In short, there are a lot of long-term and short-term benefits to getting active, so start somewhere and then find an activity or activities that not only get you moving but also bring you enjoyment.

CHAPTER VI:
Sleep, Rest & Relaxation

The Role of Sleep

Sleep is when the body enters an altered state of consciousness and shuts down all of the physical and mental work. When we're sleeping, our body recuperates. Our bodies need this time to stay healthy. Too much exercise can be damaging if we aren't allowing our bodies to recover as well. When we don't get enough sleep, it can impact our day-to-day functioning, leaving us feeling tired and irritable. Healthy sleep allows the body to boost immunity and reduce stress. Insufficient sleep can be a contributing factor to more severe conditions. Our bodies will crave more sugar and refined carbohydrates to compensate for the lack of sleep. Lack of sleep also increases stress hormones such as cortisol which kills brain cells in the memory. Sleep deprivation also affects the mood center in the brain, called the hippocampus. Sleep is good medicine. When we sleep well, it keeps us healthier.

Sleep and Diabetes

A good night's sleep is important for diabetes and overall health. Adequate sleep can help regulate appetite, mood, hormones, energy, and blood sugar. If blood sugar levels are high, someone with diabetes may have to use the restroom more frequently in the middle of the night. Insufficient sleep is also related to insulin resistance, trouble with weight loss, increased blood pressure, and an increased risk of anxiety and depression. To compensate for the lack of sleep, o

Treatment for sleep problems will depend on the underlying cause. If high blood sugar is to blame, lifestyle changes to improve glycemic control may be the first step for improving sleep. Some steps for improving sleep include:

- **Taking medication properly** – Always take medications as the doctor and pharmacist have prescribed. This is because some medications require an empty stomach to work, others cause drowsiness and should be taken before bed, and others might have stimulants that will keep you up at night if you take them too late in the day. Be sure you are clear about your doctor and pharmacist's guidance on taking your medications.

- **Eating a balanced and nutritious diet** – There's a connection between a healthy diet and sleep. Diets that are low in fiber and high in fat may decrease the amount of sleep, and as mentioned previously, excess sugar could also cause the need to use the restroom more often throughout the night. It is recommended to consume a diet high in fiber with fresh fruits and veggies, whole grains, and low-fat proteins. Also, look for foods high in Vitamin B, believed to help regulate melatonin.

- **Correcting vitamin deficiencies** – People who need vitamin B-12 deficiency may experience symptoms of peripheral neuropathy, which can impact sleep. Peripheral neuropathy results from damage to the nerves outside the brain and spinal cord; symptoms could manifest as weakness, numbness, and pain, usually in the hands and feet. Folate (vitamin B-9), Magnesium, and Iron deficiency have been linked to restless legs syndrome. Correcting a known vitamin deficiency may help if these symptoms affect your sleep.

- **Limiting caffeine and alcohol** – It is recommended to avoid caffeine and alcohol for at least 4 hours before going to bed because caffeine is a stimulant and may make it harder to fall asleep and stay asleep. Alcohol, on the other hand, may help you fall asleep but can disrupt sleep later. Sleep after drinking alcohol is linked to more frequent awakenings, night sweats, bad dreams, and headaches, thus causing less quality sleep.

- **Natural Remedies** – Additional remedies that promote better quality sleep include:

  - **Melatonin** - a hormone that our brains produce in response to darkness, which helps with the timing of circadian rhythms (or natural/internal clock). Taking natural melatonin supplements before bed can stimulate the natural production of melatonin in our brains. Melatonin has also been known to help lower glucose and blood pressure over time, adding benefits for people with diabetes.

  - **Herbal Tea** - Herbal tea can be made from edible herbs or plants. That said, there are various natural herbs known to help improve sleep and promote relaxation. According to the Sleep Foundation, if you want to improve your sleep, try one of these herbal teas (or a combination): Valerian Root, Chamomile, Lavender, Lemon Balm, or Magnolia Bark.

  - **CBD** - Cannabidiol (CBD) is a newer remedy believed to help control blood sugar, reduce stress and anxiety, and boost cardiovascular health, all of which are important for people with diabetes. Some studies even claim that CBD could help prevent diabetes.

Benefits of A Good Night's Sleep

Good sleep is connected with boosting the immune system for fighting off illness and is also linked to overall heart health. Sleep deprivation also leads to a hormone imbalance that usually leads to more sleep deprivation, which then becomes a vicious cycle.

- **Sleep Helps Fight Illness** – Sleep is essential to help attack viruses that enter the body. When we don't get good sleep, it inhibits cytokine production, reducing the body's ability to combat diseases. When you don't get enough sleep, irregular immune system activity can cause inflammation. This can ultimately lead to chronic inflammation, which increases the risk of many health conditions like ulcers, dementia, and heart disease, to name a few.

- **Sleep and Heart Health** – According to some research, more than 80% of cardiovascular events have been linked to poor sleep habits and routines. When we sleep, the body works hard to repair damage to our bodies. This damage can be from stress or harmful things we've been exposed to during the day. Sleep helps the mind and body relax and recover from the day. When we are sleep deprived, our bodies release stress hormones. Stress can make you act out of fear or make rash decisions. Chronic stress can also hurt the heart over time. Additionally, poor sleep can affect the heart indirectly by influencing food choices. Lack of sleep increases food cravings and gravitation to less heart-healthy foods. Unhealthy foods are more likely to develop high blood pressure and increase the risk of developing heart disease.

- **Poor sleep and food choices** affect the development of hormones that affect metabolism and sugar levels. This increases the risk of developing type 2 diabetes and can affect our mood, energy levels, and mental function.

- **Weight and Balance** – A good night's sleep allows the body to recuperate and maintain physical abilities. Poor sleep disrupts the balance of ghrelin and leptin, two of the many hormones regulating body weight. People who sleep less are more likely to be overweight or obese. Getting the proper amount of good sleep can help maintain those hormones needed to control appetite and body weight. Sleep deprivation can also lead to short-term balance problems called postural instability. So not only can lack sleep affect overall weight, but it can also affect how the body carries and balances itself. This combination can lead to falls and injuries.

- **Memory and Alertness** – The proper amount of sleep helps the body feel energized and alert. We can stay focused and get things done with a good night's sleep. It's also easier to exercise when we're alert and energetic. Rest also appears to play a significant role in memory consolidation. During sleep, your brain makes connections. It links events, feelings, and sensory input to form memories. Additionally, sleep can affect execution functions which involve complex thinking like problem-solving, planning, and making decisions.

Overall, sleep is a full-circle ingredient to overall health. When we lack sleep, we risk causing hormonal imbalances that have many direct and indirect effects. Let's take care of ourselves and start with a good night of rest.

The Role of Rest and Relaxation

Sleep and rest are two different things, but both are equally important to our mental, emotional, and physical health. Rest involves the whole being, not just the body. It is a state in which the body is relaxed from the stresses that come with the everyday routine. It is an activity that people should do frequently to regain energy and a refreshed mindset. Prioritizing rest and relaxation can improve the quality of sleep. That said, it is essential to prioritize adequate rest, relaxation, and sleep in everyday life.

Rest can be hard to define because it can look different for everyone. Rest can be any behavior aimed at increasing overall well-being. It can be active, like going for a walk and clearing the mind. It can also be passive, like sitting outside or meditating.

If left untreated for too long, stress can cause many harmful conditions like chest pain, headaches, digestive issues, anxiety, depression, changes in sexual desire, and inability to focus. It may seem insignificant to skip adding rest and relaxation to our daily routines, but doing so is harmful to overall wellbeing.

Deep Breathing for Relaxation

Deep breathing is essential for relaxation. Enjoy the fresh air! So, what is deep breathing? Deep breathing also comes by the name of diaphragmatic breathing, abdominal breathing, belly breathing, and paced respiration. When we breathe deeply, the air comes in through the nose, fills the lungs, and the lower belly rises. Deep breathing helps to fight damage from chronic inflammation. Science studies have shown that chronic, low-grade inflammation can become a silent killer contributing to cardiovascular disease, cancer, type 2 diabetes, and more. Breathing is essential to our lives. Deep breathing definitely helps me reduce stress and to sleep better.

CHAPTER VII:
Space

What Does "Space" Really Mean?

Every healthy relationship needs space from time to time, but what does giving someone (or ourselves) space really mean? Having uninterrupted time to ourselves allows us to pay closer attention to our emotions, process thoughts, and focus on our own needs. We all need a little extra space from time to time. When we give ourselves the time and environment to think and process our emotions, we reduce the likelihood that we'll lash out at our loved ones. Overall, space provides the ability for us to gain emotional clarity, an opportunity to take care of our individual needs, and fills our need for a sense of individuality and self-perseverance.

We need space for ourselves and our loved ones. It feels good to relax and enjoy that quiet time by ourselves. Even my garden needs space. This year I just threw my sunflower seeds back in the dirt, and they grew like crazy; it looked like a jungle. I found time to pull out the old ones, and now the new flowers are more beautiful and vibrant. Now my backyard looks good.

A close relationship with a healthy space can be a beautiful thing. When you're deeply involved with someone, you can give each other companionship and support life's challenges together, but you also need to provide each other with space at times. We shouldn't feel guilty about asking our loved ones for space, and we shouldn't feel anxious when our loved ones request some space from us.

Personal Space

When talking about personal space, there are two primary types. First, the direct distance between us. Every person has a margin of safety and can maintain it with others, also known as "personal space" or our "bubble." We have that distance to avoid awkward or uncomfortable situations with strangers, but also a sign of respect for others. The second is the physical, private space we create for ourselves. This could be a room or office where we can get some alone time. It could be a bathroom designed and decorated for relaxation and self-care.

It is essential to create your own space for "me" time. Having our own space for alone time benefits our mental health and well-being. Having a physical space and creating boundaries for ourselves gives us energy, stimulates creativity, and, most importantly, helps us relax and calm down. It offers a place of respite from a crazy world.

Maintaining space in our lives is important for romantic relationships, friendships, connections with co-workers, work environments, and more. Here are some ways that we can prioritize our individuality and space within all areas of life.

- **Strong and Open Communication –** To create and maintain space in relationships, we need to learn how to communicate openly with our loved ones. We need to be able to discuss with them when, why, and how we may need space and time for ourselves. We also need to be honest and open for them to communicate with us when they need space. Additionally, strong communication habits allow us and our loved ones confidently express how much time is required, what activities may be needed, or what support is needed.

- **Set Boundaries –** We can set boundaries for ourselves, but deciding when and how we need space from others is very important. It is okay to choose when you are in a particular space that it is dedicated to specific activities. For example: If you work from home, and you're at your desk, then that means you're at the office for work, and loved ones around the house should respect that and know not to bother you. Another example could be understanding when you're emotionally or mentally tapped and need time alone to process and recuperate. It's okay to recognize these signals and ask our loved ones to leave us alone for the evening to read a book or enjoy a creative hobby. Create and set boundaries, and once we communicate these to our loved ones, we can hold them accountable for giving us space. We should also learn what our loved ones' boundaries are and learn to adhere to and respect their boundaries.

- **Broaden Your Support System –** It is important for us to have a system of relationships. We should always nurture all connections. While having a romantic life partner can provide excellent companionship, it's also essential to maintain relationships with friends and family. It is crucial to broaden our support system because we may need different people to talk with or help through various situations we will encounter throughout our lives.

Giving Our Loved Ones Space

If a loved one asks for space, we should not be upset or jump to conclusions. It doesn't mean that they don't love us or don't want to be around us. It means they need time to feed other areas of their lives or may need some time for themselves to be able to recharge.

When we step back and allow the ones we love time and space, we give them the ability to indulge in things that make them happy, the freedom for self-care, regain control over themselves, and provide a stronger sense of self. Additionally, when we step back and allow them to have space, it can boost their self-confidence and empower them to be their best self. Most importantly, though, we show them that we trust them. We trust that they care about us and know that we care about them - enough to give them space away from us.

So, how do we give our loved ones space without losing our connection with them? Here's a general guide:

- **Ask how much time they need for themselves** – Knowing how much time they need can help ease any anxiety or nervousness around losing our loved one and knowing when it is okay to reach back out or reconnect. Find out if they need time to read a book this evening or a few days to evaluate and get control of some things causing stress in their life. This is a great way to calm our own nerves, but it also validates their feelings and needs for space.

- **Ask what they need and find out what space means for them** – It might be physical space for them to be alone to do a particular activity, or maybe they need time regularly (i.e., one night a week to be on their own). They could also be referring to needing emotional or mental space. Some people have a habit of trying to fix their loved ones' problems and might need their loved ones to let them figure something out on their own. Knowing what they need for space gives us the information we need to give our loved ones the proper space.

- **Communicate, Communicate, Communicate** – Although we may be hurt by the request or want to know more about their needs, it is important not to ask for an explanation. They do not need to validate why they need space. Instead, we should show them gratitude. We should thank them for communicating and letting us know that they need space. Next, we should let them know we're available and trust them to reach out.

- **Honor Their Request** – Once the boundaries and needs have been communicated, it's time to give them their space. Avoid reaching out and checking on them before the agreed limits.

- **Encourage Regular Moments of Space** – Give them time to do what they need to do, suggest they spend time with their friends or family, suggest an activity they enjoy doing, and set aside time to do their favorite thing on a regular basis. Suggest new events or activities they may enjoy.

- **Do Your Own Thing** – Sometimes, we can get too involved in our relationships and friendships and neglect our own interests. We must also find time to do our own "things," which gives our loved ones the liberty to do the same. When they see that we're taking time to do things on our own, they will be more inclined to take time and space for themselves. So, get out there and connect with friends and family! Get involved with something challenging, start volunteering, or add reading to the routine.

CHAPTER VIII:
Let's Be Good to Ourselves

Part I is an overall explanation of why good health is vital to what our body needs. Our mind and body need stimulation, joy, self-care, a positive attitude, space, proper sleep, rest and relaxation, and proper nutrients. We also need a strong desire to take good care of our health, which is the first step in healthy living. We should include activities that will bring joy and stimulate our brains, like playing with our children, family, and friends. Learning new things, reading, and writing also help to stimulate our brains and improve our decision-making. Staying fit physically, emotionally, socially, mentally, and spiritually are all very important to our health. Practicing healthy habits daily will improve our physical and mental health. Gratitude and being thankful will help us become good people and improve our health. Be kind to everyone, especially to yourself.

The more we learn about health, the easier it is to take good care of our bodies. Taking time to take good care of our health is a must. It is necessary to be able to take good care of others. Health is something we ignore till it is too late. That is why it is so important to me that I share my passion for healthy living. Spending time with myself and with my thoughts has restored my good health. I continually choose to let positive thoughts occupy my mind, and negative thoughts disappear.

I used to be a shallow breather. When I started going to the gym, I saw a bunch of older women gathering to take up a space to exercise together, and they were having a good time. They had positive attitudes, which created a happy and healthy atmosphere. They were looking forward to a healthy, vibrant life ahead of them. I was thinking about some of those older people that are cranky, drinking alcohol, and smoking. All they talk about are their frustrations and sharing about their illnesses and their medications. Obviously, their health choices aren't leading to a healthy lifestyle or a vibrant life ahead. See the difference? I sure can! I learned that people with a positive attitude usually have healthier habits; they may eat healthy food, exercise regularly, rarely smoke, and drink less alcohol. They may experience less stress and see good even in a bad situation.

Being active is the best way to stay in shape. Not everybody enjoys exercising. Playing with your pet, children, and anybody you can spend time with will be helpful. Gardening, doing errands for somebody, and doing your chores are the best choices. Walking is very good for any age. Regular physical activities may improve and maintain strength as we age.

Healthy sleep will help us feel energized and focused. There is nothing better than getting up refreshed. Rest and relaxation are vital for our concentration and may reduce stress, improve mood and get better sleep. Deep breathing is one way I enjoy my relaxation time.

Space is where I can create, express my thoughts, then put them to work. I create my life from my thoughts, the words I speak, and what I believe. Things get so tricky when I am so busy all the time. Being alone to think and recuperate from my busy life can be very good for my physical and mental health. I can enjoy the rest of the day after I enjoy that space by myself.

Our bodies don't need boredom, negative thoughts, neglect of our health, frustration, inadequate sleep, physical, mental, and emotional stress, and the list goes on. There are no excuses for being bored. There are a lot of people around and a lot of activities to choose from available to us. Let's enjoy all those blessings. Changing our thoughts to more enthusiastic and optimistic will produce joy and energy. Let's be good to ourselves and live a healthy lifestyle.

Part II:
THE EFFECTS OF HEALTH, HAPPINESS & STRESS

CHAPTER IX:
Health & Wellness

Good Health & Wellness

Good health is a crucial component of human happiness and well-being. It also contributes to prosperity, wealth, and even economic progress. Studies have shown that healthy populations are more productive, save more, and often live longer.

What is the meaning of wellness? It is the quality of being in good health through pursuing activities, choices, and lifestyles that leads to overall health. Overall, wellness is the active process of becoming more aware and making choices toward a healthy, purpose-driven, and fulfilled life. We're talking about more than just being free from illness. It is a dynamic process that reflects change and growth. Wellness is a primary factor in good physical and mental health. Mental health and physical health are so closely linked. That is, problems in one area can impact the other and vice-versa. Overall, wellness is the act of practicing healthy habits daily to attain better physical outcomes so that instead of just surviving, we're thriving.

So, how does wellness improve health? Wellness includes social connectedness, exercise, nutrition, sleep, and mindfulness. Each one has an impact on our physical and mental health. By making a simple and healthy daily basis, we will be on our way toward reducing stress, having positive social interaction, and achieving optimal wellness. Health and wellness go hand in hand; we can't have one without the other. But what is the primary difference between health and wellness? Health is the goal, and wellness is the active process of achieving that goal.

Benefits of Good Health & Wellness

Good health and wellness include a variety of aspects of our lives, from exercise and activity to hygiene, eating a balanced diet, mental wellness, and much more. While the effects of bad habits are often shoved in our faces, the benefits of healthy habits aren't always as widely discussed (at least in an understandable way). So, let's break some of this down!

- **Fight Disease** – One of the more important benefits of good health includes fighting off disease and health complications. Conditions such as cancer, diabetes, and heart failure, have all been linked to poor health choices and a sedentary lifestyle. Eating a balanced and nutritious diet, rich in fruits and veggies, equips the body with the fiber and antioxidants needed to flush toxins and keep the cells healthy. Additionally, eating plenty of fiber and getting enough prebiotics will also help prevent digestive disease. Pair these eating habits with regular exercise for a powerful disease-fighting combination.

- **Self-Confidence** – Self-confidence is part of good health, but where does it come from? It comes first from not neglecting the small, daily disciplines. It's about feeling good about ourselves and knowing that we did our best at the end of the day. When working on writing a letter, it is knowing it's the best letter you could write. You can use the tools and knowledge available. At the end of those days, when you feel good about yourself, self-confidence begins to rise.

  Willingness to do whatever it takes to achieve your goals is necessary. If you must read more books and learn more, you must do whatever it takes to reach your goals. Whatever allows you to rise above your current circumstances and encourages you to keep going. Self-confidence and overcoming circumstances empower you to persist and achieve your goals.

  We also gain confidence when we work out regularly. Walking, running, swimming, or dancing. It may be hard for some. However, the challenges and pain become worth it in time. The more confidence we build up mentally and physically, the more we believe in ourselves to take on.

- **Personal Hygiene** – Personal hygiene is also a part of good health. Practicing good hygiene influences a person's body image. The main principle of good hygiene is keeping the external body clean and properly groomed. It involves just a few tasks, but we need to stay clean as it helps minimize the risk of getting sick. Good hygiene doesn't have to mean stocking up on expensive products. If we want to take care of our bodies, there are many natural and inexpensive ways to do this. Ancient secret #1: In the olden days, they used cornstarch for face powder. To this day, I still use cornstarch as my face powder. I remember when I was a kid, my mom would pat cornstarch all over our bodies after a bath to avoid heat rashes because it is so hot in the Philippines. Taking a shower regularly, brushing your teeth, and trimmed nails will be sufficient for having good personal hygiene. Looking well-groomed, clean, and tidy will improve your overall health.

- **Mood and Brain Health** – Positive changes occur in the brain when we exercise. Working out allows our bodies to circulate blood and oxygen more efficiently. This helps create new brain cells and a stronger connection between the cells that communicate. These effects help boost our mood as well as improve our memory. Additionally, regular exercise has been connected to reducing stress, anger, anxiety, and depression. So when we include regular activity into our routine, we improve our mental wellness and create changes in the brain to boost our overall mood.

- **Physical Benefits** – First, let's talk about a healthy gut and internal organs. The stomach contains many different bacteria, both good and bad. There is a proper balance between the good and the bad bacteria, which only occurs when there are more good bacteria than bad bacteria. The naturally occurring bacteria help the body with digestion function and metabolism. There are also other good bacteria, such as those that help create vitamins B and K, which fight harmful bacteria and viruses in the body. When our gut system is off balance, it causes local inflammation. If this is not treated, it could cause larger, more systemic issues in our bodies.

  Our balanced diet should include eating fiber, fermented foods, and getting enough prebiotics and probiotics. These all work together to help the colon thrive and therefore prevent digestive issues and diseases. Exercise is also vital to a healthy gut and organs because it helps improve blood flow and prevents poor circulation. Optimized blood flow throughout the body ensures the body gets the nutrients needed from the food we eat. Blood is also the means of transportation, sending cells and hormones from one area of the body to another.

  Another physical benefit of regular exercise and wellness is maintaining a healthy weight and weight loss. A balanced diet rich in lean protein, heavy in plant-based ingredients, and high in fiber typically allows for weight loss without restricting how much can be eaten. We are more likely to stay healthy and achieve maintenance and weight loss goals when we refrain from eating sugary or overly processed foods. Additionally, working out helps burn off excess calories and eliminate excess fat. This helps reduce stress on the body, and when we maintain a healthy weight, it helps reduce the workload on our organs.

Are you in pain? We choose our pain. Let me explain. We all know brushing our teeth is essential, but we choose to skip it. Then, suddenly we have a toothache. When we are diagnosed with diabetes, we choose to go out to eat unhealthy foods and continue our sedentary lifestyle. Our kidneys will complain and start to shut down. If we have a bad kidney, then we must go through dialysis.

It is obvious when our situation needs special attention. We must follow the doctor's advice and take our medication faithfully. The point is we must sacrifice instant gratification and choose to take care of our health. Either way, we must take care of something. If we don't take care of our health now, sooner or later, we may be forced to take care of illness. I have watched my family suffer and die from diabetes. I started making my health and wellness a priority. I am that important. I'm telling you, it's not fun taking all those medications, treating those illnesses, and being in a bad mood because you're in pain. By the way, my spouse, my friends, and everybody around me enjoy my company when I am happy. I am happy because I am healthy. It is a win-win situation.

I must be aware of what I am doing before I do it. I always ask myself, "What would happen if I did this?" I know, I am weird. I talk to myself too much, but I know myself more than anybody else. Besides, there are always conflicts every time there is another person involved. If I don't know what to do or the answer, I am quick to ask for help. Learning to be aware of how I live and what I do to make myself healthy was hard at first. After a while, as I went along, I realized that I felt much better and happier. When I am healthy, I choose more wisely. That is one of the benefits of being healthy. My brain works better. My choices are better. This process does take time. Practice, practice, practice. It is worth it!

CHAPTER X:
Happiness

What is Happiness?

The Merriam-Webster dictionary definition of happiness is the state of well-being and contentment or joy. It is also described as the feeling that comes over you when you know life is good, and you can't help but smile. People often refer to it as the opposite of sadness. When people are successful, safe, or lucky, they feel happiness. The pursuit of happiness is something this country is based on, and different people feel happiness for various reasons. Whenever doing something causes happiness, people usually want to do more of it. No one has ever complained about feeling too much happiness.

Happiness is inside of you. If you don't have it, create it. It's not going to fall in your lap. You can't find it in things or people. It's within you. Happiness, in psychology, is a state of emotional well-being that a person experiences when good things happen in a specific moment or more positive evaluation of one's life and accomplishments. Happiness is the feeling of true happiness in your life and the desire to make the very best of it. It is the "thing" that can help us do our best. Happy people tend to be more successful and well-rounded in life.

Proven Benefits of Happiness

While we all strive for happiness in life, there are proven benefits of happiness that can affect physical and mental health, as well as overall well-being. First, when we are happy, we improve our heart health and lower the risk of heart disease by 13-26%. Additionally, when we are happy, we tend to reduce stress which is good for our bodies, as excess stress causes higher levels of cortisol. Cortisol is the stress hormone that can lead to several health conditions, including complications with the heart. Some studies have also shown that being happier can support a stronger immune system. Therefore, when we are happy, we have a greater ability to fight infections and diseases more effectively.

Generally, when we are happy, we are likely to make better choices regarding lifestyle and healthy habits. Happy people tend to have a greater sense of well-being, including eating more nutritious diets. These healthy habits include engaging in more physical activities and overcoming poor sleeping habits. Happiness brings joy and may help with having a healthier mind, body, and spirit.

Happiness: Techniques According to Science

Are you happy? There's a lot of teaching, seminars, articles, workshops, books, audio, and social media on how to be happy. Yet, there are still a lot of people that are unhappy. Everybody has different ways to be happy. What makes me happy might frustrate you. We can become happy even when we are going through tough times.

Some studies test and prove that happiness can be achieved, even in tough times, if we implement a few techniques and habits into our lives. Next, I will share the methods, according to science, to increase the happy hormones in our bodies. What are happy hormones, you ask? Happy hormones send a message to the brain to trigger the brain to emit emotions and feelings of happiness. These hormones travel through the bloodstream and bring signals to different parts of the body. These happy hormones can affect our stress levels, promote joy, positive feelings, love, pleasure, and more. There are four main hormones that make us happy.

- **Oxytocin** – This is a bonding hormone that causes a reduction in blood pressure and cortisol. It reduces the stress hormone norepinephrine and can induce relaxation. Some ways to increase oxytocin include enjoying aroma therapy which can help with relaxation and energy. Oxytocin levels can also spike when we ask a loved one for a hug, and when we make it a point to find the good things in every situation and interaction we encounter. Another way to increase oxytocin is to get a pet. Research has shown that petting a dog or family pet lowers the stress hormone cortisol, and the social interaction between people and their pets increases oxytocin levels.

- **Serotonin** – This hormone is a mood stabilizer. It is the chemical in the body that carries messages between nerve cells in the brain and throughout the body. Serotonin plays an essential role in body functions like mood, sleep, digestion, wound healing, and sexual desire. Lack of serotonin is thought to play a role in depression, anxiety, and other health conditions. There are a few key ways to increase our serotonin levels. The first, get more sunlight. A little sun every day (even just 10 to 15 minutes) can benefit serotonin creation and overall mood. So, get outside more! Go for a bike ride or walk around the park. Another way to increase serotonin is by working on reducing stress. Try listening to your favorite music, work on completing tasks, or enjoying physical touch with loved ones. Finally, serotonin can increase when we eat more tryptophan-containing foods. Add more eggs, turkey, cheese, and salmon to your diet. Pineapple, nuts, oats, and seeds are also good sources of tryptophan.

- **Endorphins** – These are hormones that are released when the body feels pain or stress. These hormones are produced in the brain and act as messengers in the body to help relieve pain, reduce stress, and improve mood and sense of well-being. A lack of endorphins in the system can cause symptoms of depression, anxiety, addiction or impulsive actions, sleep issues, and body aches and pains. The good news is we can boost endorphins through regular exercise. Endorphins can also be released when we eat or get a massage. Endorphins are also released during sex. Endorphins promote the release of dopamine, another neurotransmitter that affects our mood.

- **Dopamine** – This hormone, also known as the pleasure chemical or "feel good" hormone, plays a role in many essential body functions, which include memory, movement, motivation, and more. This is the hormone that gives us a sense of pleasure. It is also the hormone that rewards us when we're doing things we need to do, which gives us the motivation to keep doing something. When we do something pleasurable, the brain releases a large amount of dopamine. Thus, we feel good and seek to do more of the thing that produced those pleasant feelings. When dopamine levels are too high or too low, this is associated with conditions such as Parkinson's disease, ADHD, and addiction.

These happy hormones help with my healthy living habits. When I am happy, I am healthy. It works for me. Inspiration helps me to become successful, happy, and loving. I create my own future. It will not happen if I sit down and do nothing. I must work on it, and it always brings me joy.

CHAPTER XI:
Stress

The Meaning of Stress

Stress is a state of demanding circumstances in which our body responds to mental pressure. Stress is a natural reaction to life experiences and is often a psychological and physical response. Stress triggers can range from everyday things like work responsibilities to our response to significant life events, like losing a job or receiving a health diagnosis. Stress is also associated with chronic inflammation, which can significantly impact overall health. Cortisol, as mentioned before, is known as the "stress hormone." Lowering the cortisol level in our bodies will help us to stay healthy and live longer.

How Stress Affects the Body

Certain types of stress are beneficial, but long-term stress makes life more challenging and can have a negative effect on our health.

 Now, there is such a thing as good stress. Good stress is beneficial because it makes us work harder and better. It helps us learn healthy coping techniques and skills. With good stress, we are able to accomplish goals and complete tasks. In situations of potential danger, the body can release hormones like cortisol, increase heart rate, and prepare the muscles to respond.

Long-term stress, however, is not good for our bodies. It is uncomfortable and damaging to the body and mind. Prolonged stress often causes difficulty falling or staying asleep, frequent headaches, anxiety, depression, and irritability. Stress can also affect core systems throughout the body, including:

- **Digestive System** – When under stress, the liver makes more glucose than the body can manage. This excess glucose can cause diarrhea, bloating, or constipation.

- **Central Nervous System** – Being anxious is one of the most well-known effects of stress on the body. The brain releases two different stress hormones, cortisol and adrenaline, which increase blood flow throughout the body to organs and muscles.

- **Cardiovascular System** – When there is prolonged stress, the heart rate increases. When we are stressed out, it can increase the risk of a heart attack or a stroke.

- **Respiratory System** – When under stress, it also causes breathing to increase. This is the body's response to distribute more oxygen throughout the body. Anxiety constricts that flow even though breathing is increased.

- **Reproductive System** – Stress often causes a decrease in sexual desire. Men can have interrupted sperm production or dysfunction. For women, prolonged stress can cause changes to the menstrual cycle that make it heavier, lighter, or irregular.

- **Immune System** – When the body is stressed, it can make us more susceptible to becoming sick. It also lengthens the time the body can recover from illness or injury.

- **Musculoskeletal System** – Chronic stress causes the muscles to go into a constant state of tension that causes aches and pains. It may eventually lead to other injuries or stress-related disorders.

How to Reduce Stress

If we're constantly feeling stressed, it can be hard to recognize that we are indeed under stress. Recognizing the feeling of stress is the first step in dealing with it. We think we're fine, but when we don't allow ourselves to be stressed and work through it, then it just increases. So, don't keep hustling without drinking water, having something to eat, and taking breaks to shake it out. We also need to recognize what causes us stress and ensure we avoid the cortisol build-up in our bodies.

One of the leading causes of high levels of cortisol can be caused by psychological stress. So, one of the first things we can do is get control of our psychological stresses. Start by focusing on the good in situations and not dwelling on the negative or obstacles. We can also avoid high cortisol levels when we stop overeating, avoid sugary foods, and focus more on a plant-based diet. Also, lifting weights, even a light weight, can help the body burn off excess cortisol.

If we are stressed out all the time, or more frequently, we will speed up our bodies' aging process. Many studies have shown that people with a high level of stress tend to be chronically ill and even have an acceleration of gray hair. That's a fact, not just a myth. We really do get older if we have too much stress.

CHAPTER XII:
Detox

Detox is a process in which one abstains from harmful or unwanted substances for an extended period of time to rid the body of toxic or unhealthy substances. It typically implies using supplements or following a special diet that claims to rid the body of toxins to promote weight loss or improve health. While detox diets have their appeal, the body is equipped to handle toxins and other unwanted substances naturally.

That said, there are ways you can help detox your body without needing fad diets or expensive supplements.

- **Get More Sleep:** Poor sleep has been linked to short and long-term health consequences. Stress, anxiety, high blood pressure, obesity, and type 2 diabetes are connected to lack of sleep or poor sleep. The body must get adequate and quality sleep every night to support health and natural detoxification. With sleep deprivation, the body does not have time to remove toxic waste by-products that accumulate throughout the day.

- **Stay Active:** Regular exercise reduces the risk of many diseases, including type 2 diabetes, heart disease, and high blood pressure. Exercise helps to reduce inflammation. While some inflammation helps when recovering from an infection or healing wounds, too much inflammation can weaken the body's system and actually promote disease. With exercise, we can reduce inflammation which can help the body's systems, including the detoxification system.

- **Reduce Sugar and Salt Intake:** High consumption of sugar and highly processed foods has been considered to cause obesity, heart disease, cancer, diabetes, and other chronic illnesses. These conditions can hinder the body's ability to detoxify by harming the organs with these essential roles. Consumption of excessive sugar can cause fatty liver, limiting liver functions. Consuming too much salt can cause the body to retain excess fluid. When we consume too much salt and not enough water, the body releases a hormone that is an antidiuretic. This antidiuretic prevents urination, hindering the body's ability to detoxify. We can eliminate excess water retention by increasing water intake, reducing sodium, and eating potassium-rich foods. Increasing the consumption of potassium-rich foods can counterbalance some of sodium's effects on the body.

- **Limit Alcohol:** Excessive drinking can severely damage the liver by causing fat build-up and inflammation. When this happens to the liver, it cannot function properly to filter waste and other toxins from the body. Limiting, or abstaining from, alcohol is one of the best ways to keep the body's detoxification processes moving smoothly.

- **Drink More Water:** Keeping the body properly hydrated is vital for detoxification. Water has many functions, including aiding digestion and nutrient absorption and detoxifying the body by removing waste. Water transports waste products and toxins to be removed from the body. These toxins and waste products could be harmful if build-up occurs in the blood.

- **Antioxidant-rich Food and Prebiotics:** Antioxidants protect cells against damage caused by molecules known as free radicals. Oxidative stress results from the excessive production of free radicals. Eating foods rich in antioxidants helps counter oxidative stress caused by free radicals. Antioxidants can also oppose the effects of toxins that increase the risk of diseases impacting the detoxification system. Gut health is essential to keeping the detoxification system healthy. Good gut health starts with prebiotics, a type of fiber that feeds good bacteria in the gut. Eating food with high content of prebiotics helps the good bacteria produce nutrients that are beneficial for health. Eating antioxidant-rich foods and foods with a high content of prebiotics can keep the immune and detoxification systems strong.

Certain dietary changes and lifestyle practices can help reduce toxins load and support the body's detoxification system. Other helpful tips for detoxification include:

- Eating foods high in sulphur, like onions and broccoli, enhance the excretion of heavy metals like cadmium. Eating sulphur-rich foods aids the function of glutathione. Glutathione is an antioxidant involved in detoxification.

- Add flavor with cilantro, which has properties that aid in reducing swelling and enhance the excretion of toxins like lead and chemicals.

- Switch to natural cleaning products and body care products. Natural cleaning products such as vinegar and baking soda can reduce exposure to toxic chemicals. Also, choosing natural body care products like deodorants, makeup moisturizers, and shampoo can minimize exposure to chemicals.

When I learned about this, it was excellent information. Come to find out, I had been detoxing unnecessarily. I had already been eating healthy and following an antioxidant diet. This information will save me time, money, and effort. I no longer spend money or time on detox supplements. Instead, I am enjoying learning and detoxing naturally.

CHAPTER XIII:
Prioritize Health

We must change our habits to healthier ones. As I mentioned in Part I, it is valuable in our daily lives. Part II, it is just as important to prioritize our valuable health before it is too late. There are claims that people are now living longer, but I see many more family members and friends die early or may be avoiding death but they just exist.

I have a cousin that has been bedridden for twenty years. Somebody must take care of her because of her illness. Another example is my husband's friend, who has been bedridden for just as long as my cousin has. If life is just to lay there and barely move, it is not really considered living but rather simply existing. My definition of living is moving and still enjoying things in life. Optimal health is living our best life.

You have the best health and enjoy life to the fullest. It is different for everybody. My best life might not be your best life. Stress will definitely ruin optimal health. Simple living may eliminate some of the unnecessary stress. A little stress is good for us. It gives us a spark. Stress challenges us to make us work harder and better. Too much stress will lead to chronic illness.

A positive attitude will improve our mood. People enjoy being around others that are joyful and in good spirits. It also improves our health in the process. We should approach every situation and challenge with a positive mental attitude. We should be optimistic and enthusiastic but don't give in to negativity. When we stay positive, it uplifts others as well.

Self-love is having a high regard for our own happiness and well-being. It helps us take good care of ourselves and others. When we neglect ourselves, we become ill and irritated that we cannot care for ourselves and others. Being in good health makes us better parents, partners, friends, workers, and leaders. Because we love ourselves, we eat healthy, stop what we are doing and take a break, get a good night's sleep, pray, and meditate. We do things that are important to us. Our cup is always full. Self-love gives us the courage to be kind to ourselves, leading to better mental, physical, and emotional health.

Learning and doing new things has excitedly and drastically improved my life. It is a blessing to meet new people. I am enjoying myself, and I am learning from them. Change has given me experiences and opportunities to enjoy life to the fullest. It has helped me become healthier because I learned to make better decisions and choices. I am eating healthier, exercising, and choosing wholesome activities.

Enjoy life. Do something you enjoy and love to do. Keep the company of people who like the same activities you enjoy. When you do this, it will eliminate arguing with those around you. Doing nothing is boring and bad for our health. Remember, "Health is Wealth." Take care now! Be happy.

Part III:
NUTRITION, SUPPLEMENTS & RECIPES

CHAPTER XIV: Nutrition Guide

Nutrition Elements

Natural and whole foods are far better for our health and well-being. Our bodies don't need, and can't process as well, chemicals, processed foods, additives, or preservatives. Manufacturers must add chemicals to food to make it taste better and last longer. Those chemicals slowly ruin our health, so It takes a long time before the damage to our health really becomes noticeable. By then, it's usually too late.

I am often asked what I include in my diet and routine to help with my health. I am also often asked how I have avoided diseases and health issues that many of my family members died from or are currently suffering from. Here are some nutritional elements that I have added to my routine and recommend to others.

- **Apple Cider Vinegar (ACV)** – Apple Cider Vinegar is the product of a two-part process in which crushed apples are exposed to yeast. This addition of yeast ferments the sugars and turns them into alcohol. Then bacteria are added, which further ferments the alcohol into acetic acid. Researchers believe this acid is responsible for the health benefits of ACV. Apple Cider Vinegar is believed to be suitable for:
    - **Improved Satiety and Weight Loss:** Some studies have shown that ACV might make you want to eat less because of the compound from the fermented apple that suppresses your appetite. Drinking 2 tbsp of ACV with a glass of water during meals may reduce sugar crashes and stabilize blood sugar levels.
    - **Boost Skin Health:** Apple cider vinegar is naturally acidic and has antimicrobial properties, which can help improve the skin barrier and prevent infections. It has been linked to preventing dandruff, improving acne, and fading aging spots. That said, please consult your doctor or dermatologist before using, as ACV can also irritate the skin if misused.
    - **Reduce Risk of Infection and Kill Bacteria:** The primary substance in vinegar, acetic acid, kills harmful bacteria and prevents them from multiplying. This helps reduce the risk of infection, but ACV can also be useful in cleaning and as a disinfectant.

- o **Ease Digestion and Bloating:** Since ACV is naturally acidic, it can help raise acid levels in the stomach to aid digestion. This could also prevent gas and bloating, which are often caused by slow digestion. As mentioned previously, since ACV is an antimicrobial substance, it can also help kill bacteria in the stomach and intestines.

  - o **Relieving Leg Cramps:** Though Apple Cider Vinegar is acidic and may not contain many vitamins, it is high in potassium, which makes it an excellent natural remedy for leg cramps.

- **Avocado –** Avocados are an incredibly nutritious fruit. They are a good source of healthy fat, fiber, and vitamins. Avocados contain antioxidants and anti-inflammatory compounds that may help reduce heart disease. The avocado's high potassium and magnesium content helps keep blood pressure healthy. Other benefits of avocado include:

  - o **Boost Nutrient Absorption:** Once we consume valuable nutrients, the body must adequately absorb them from the digestive tract and into the bloodstream. Many of the much-needed nutrients are fat-soluble, meaning we must consume them with fat to receive the full spectrum of benefits. Avocado, being full of healthy fats, helps improve nutrient absorption from the avocado itself and other healthy foods.

  - o **Eyes & Brain:** Avocado contains the carotenoid and antioxidant lutein which is critical to eye health. Lutein gets deposited in the retina to help filter out harmful light and protect against free radicals. As a source of healthy unsaturated fats, avocados may support the brain by lowering blood pressure.

  - o **Heart Health:** Avocado contains fiber, potassium, and magnesium. All of which help lower blood pressure and cholesterol to help keep the bloodstream healthy.

  - o **Hair and Skin:** Avocado is full of monounsaturated fats, and vitamins C and E, nutrients that help improve skin tone and maintain moisture. Avocados also contain an antioxidant that guards against damage from sun exposure.

- **Berries –** Berries are often referred to as one of the healthiest foods on earth. They are nutrient-rich, and one of the top sources of vitamins and minerals. Berries are loaded with antioxidants and high in fiber. They are so nutrient-rich, studies show they may help reduce the risk of many age-related conditions. Benefits of berries may include:

- o **Blood Sugar & Insulin Response:** Berries may improve blood sugar and insulin levels when consumed with high-carb foods or included in smoothies. Research studies have found that adding berries (primarily blueberries and strawberries) to a daily diet can positively impact blood sugar levels and help increase insulin sensitivity. Eating berries high in anthocyanins (mostly blueberries and strawberries) can also help people keep weight off.

- o **Cholesterol, Heart & Arteries:** Berries, primarily black raspberries and strawberries, have been shown to lower LDL cholesterol levels and help prevent it from becoming oxidized. This may reduce the risk of heart disease. Additionally, black raspberries and strawberries have been shown in studies to help lower cholesterol, even in people who are obese or have metabolic syndromes. In addition to lowering cholesterol, berries can help improve the function of the arteries. The endothelial cells line the blood vessels, control blood pressure, prevent clotting, and many other processes. These cells are damaged by excessive inflammation and prevent proper operation. When this occurs, it is a significant risk factor for heart disease. Berries have been found to improve the function of these endothelial cells, thus lowering the risk of heart disease and heart attack.

- o **Increased Satiety and Weight Management:** Berries are high in fiber, including soluble fiber. The soluble fiber slows down the movement of food in the digestive tract, reducing hunger and producing a feeling of fullness—both of which may help with calorie intake and weight management.

- o **Fight Inflammation:** The antioxidants in berries have strong anti-inflammatory properties. While inflammation is the body's mechanism for defense against injury or infections, excessive and long-term inflammation can lead to conditions like diabetes and heart disease. Studies have shown that the antioxidants in berries help reduce these inflammatory markers.

- **Blue Cheese –** Blue cheese is rich in potassium, calcium, zinc, and phosphorus. It is also an excellent source of Vitamin A. Be careful with serving size because blue cheese is also high in sodium. Although Blue cheese is higher in saturated fats than healthy fats, it still provides a good serving of unsaturated fats, which can protect the heart. Some potential health benefits of blue cheese include:

- o **Bone Health:** One serving of blue cheese contains 10% of the recommended daily calcium intake. Calcium is responsible for bone density and strengthening of the bones. Keep in mind though, that calcium is not easily absorbed without Vitamin D. Blue cheese does not contain much Vitamin D, so it is recommended to pair blue cheese with other foods that are sources of Vitamin D.

  - o **Assist with Absorption of Vitamins:** As mentioned previously, many essential vitamins are fat-soluble and best consumed with foods high in fat. The fat content in blue cheese will help with the absorption of fat-soluble foods eaten with it.

  - o **Quality Protein Source:** One serving of blue cheese can provide 6 grams of protein per ounce, making it a great source of protein. The protein content of blue cheese is Casein, a milk protein that contains all nine essential amino acids. Essential amino acids assist with growth and nitrogen balance. Casein is also a slow-digesting protein, ideal for long periods without eating, like during a fast.

- **Carrots** – Carrots are a very versatile vegetable, it is well known that carrots have essentials for eye health, but there are a variety of other benefits, which may include:

  - o **Boost Immunity:** Beta-carotene, an antioxidant in carrots, is linked to eye health and also helps produce Vitamin A in the body. Vitamin A is vital to boosting the immune system and helps the body respond to intruders and regenerate new cells to stay strong.

  - o **Skin Health:** The carotenoids retinol, biotin, and lycopene are also found in carrots. These are good for the skin.

  - o **Brain Health:** Luteolin, another nutrient found in carrots, helps keep the brain healthy. Eating carrots regularly may help boost memory and prevent cognitive decline over time.

- **Chamomile Tea** – Chamomile is an ancient herb used in herbal medicine for centuries. It has many soothing and therapeutic properties and can be used in various ways, most commonly in essential oils and herbal tea. Historically, chamomile has been used for its preventative and curative properties and for a variety of ailments. Today, it is most associated with sleep and relaxation, but there are a few other benefits to a daily cup of chamomile tea.

  - o **Anxiety and Sleep:** Chamomile is a mild sedative that can help physically and mentally calm. It is known for its relaxing and soothing properties, making it an excellent option for reducing stress and anxiety. It is also a common recommendation if you need help falling asleep at night.

- o **Anti-inflammatory and Anti-allergy Properties:** Chamomile is often used as a natural antihistamine as it has properties that prevent the discharge of histamines that trigger allergic reactions throughout the body. One or two daily cups of chamomile tea (sweetened with local honey) can provide immunity to many common allergens. Chamomile also has anti-inflammatory properties and has been used for chronic inflammatory conditions like arthritis.

  Aids with Lowering Blood Sugar and Diabetes: Some studies have found that chamomile tea can help lower blood sugar in people with diabetes. It is not a viable substitute for diabetes medications, but it may be a helpful supplement to existing treatments. Other studies have found that consistent consumption of chamomile tea might aid in preventing blood sugar from increasing, which suggests that chamomile could improve diabetes outcomes.

- **Chia Seeds** – Chia seeds are an ancient superfood, primarily in Aztec and Mayan diets. It is a concentrated protein source and is also rich in fiber, which helps keep the body full and energized. Chia seeds also contain antioxidants, minerals, and omega-3 fatty acids. These nutrients play a role in supporting multiple body functions and systems. Chia seeds can be added to baked goods or sprinkled on cereal or savory dishes. Chia seeds expand into a gel when added to liquid, making them an excellent option for thickening sauces. Despite their tiny size, chia seeds have many potential health benefits:

  - o **Promote Healthy Digestion & Aid in Managing Blood Sugar:** Chia seeds are packed with fiber, stimulating digestion. Chia seeds provide 40% of the daily recommended fiber intake. Fiber does not require as much energy to process because it doesn't raise blood sugar or require insulin. Diets high in fiber can slow digestion, which may improve blood sugar levels. Furthermore, chia seeds are a rich source of protein and omega-3s. This combination can help metabolic health and stabilize blood sugar levels.

  - o **Increase Energy:** The carbohydrates in chia seeds have a slower conversion time. This means that they fuel energy for the body longer. Since it takes longer to digest, nutrients are available for longer. This is why chia seeds are a common ingredient in energy and meal replacement bars.

- o **Bone Health:** Chia seeds are high in magnesium, phosphorus, calcium, and ALA. These nutrients have been linked to improved bone density. One ounce of chia seeds can contain 15 to 20 percent of the recommended daily intake of calcium.

- o **Boost Mood:** Chia seeds contain tryptophan, an amino acid that helps people feel calmer and more sedated. Tryptophan helps the brain increase the production and reception of serotonin and regulates melatonin levels. Serotonin helps relieve anxiety, and melatonin can help improve sleep.

- o **Cardiovascular Health:** Chia seeds are high in fiber and are a viable source of omega-3 fatty acids which help reduce inflammation and may reduce the risk of heart disease. Chia seeds can also help raise HDL, the healthy cholesterol, and lower LDL (bad cholesterol) in the blood. This can also help reduce the risk of heart disease.

- o **Stimulate Weight Loss:** Chia seeds are high in fiber and protein, which have been linked to aiding weight loss. The high fiber content can help facilitate the absorption of water, which makes the stomach expand and feel fuller. Fiber also aids the digestive system in running smoothly. The high-protein content may help control appetite and hunger. Adding chia seeds is unlikely to cause weight loss, but it plays a useful role in reaching a healthy weight when combined with a balanced diet and regular exercise.

- **Cilantro** – Cilantro (Coriandrum sativum L), also known as Coriander, is an herbal plant in a family of mostly aromatic flowering plants containing over three thousand species. Among this family are also carrots, celery, and parsley. Cilantro is the leaf, and Coriander is the seed of the coriander plant.   It can be used in cooking and alternative medicine. Cilantro has been linked to many health benefits, including reducing the risk of heart disease, diabetes, obesity, and seizure severity. The herb is a good source of lipids. It also contains linalool, an essential oil. The benefits of adding cilantro to a balanced diet include the following:

  - o **May Aid in Protecting Against Cancer:** It has been found that cooking with cilantro can prevent the development of HCAs, or heterocyclic amines. HCAs arise when meat is cooked at high temperatures. High consumption of HCAs has been linked to an increased risk of cancer. Researchers have also found that the herb has reduced the expression of specific genes in cancer cells, which may help cancer cells become less invasive and limit the cells from grouping together in colonies.

- o **Limit Sodium Intake:** Cilantro can add a fresh and citrusy flavor to almost any dish. It is usually added at the end as it doesn't withstand prolonged heat. Due to cilantro's flavor profile, using cilantro to flavor food may encourage people to use less salt and reduce their sodium intake.

- o **Anticonvulsant Properties:** Studies have found that cilantro may reduce the occurrence of epileptic seizures. It is thought that a component of cilantro, dodecanal, binds to a potent potassium channel referred to as the KCNQ. Dysfunction of this channel can cause brain damage or disease due to epileptic seizures. The dodecanal in cilantro binds to the KCNQ channel, which has shown the potential to help reduce the activity that causes seizures.

- o **Healthy Skin:** A study in the Journal of Medicinal Food examined the ability of coriander leaf extracts and the ability to protect against ultraviolet B damage. The results supported the potential to prevent or reduce sun damage to the skin.

- **Cinnamon** – There are many types of cinnamon around the world. It has been used as a spice for cooking and medicinal purposes for thousands of years. Cinnamon comes from the bark of various species of cinnamon trees. Possible health benefits of cinnamon include:
  - o **Loaded with Antioxidants:** Cinnamon is rich and powerful in antioxidants. It has been shown to contain more antioxidants than garlic and oregano. Antioxidants shield the body from free radicals that cause oxidative stress. Cinnamon may increase the body's ability to fight off free radicals helping to keep the body healthy and protected from disease.

  - o **Aid in Fighting Diabetes:** Cinnamon may help improve sensitivity to insulin and help lower blood sugar levels. It may also help improve metabolism, which can help the pancreas. Cinnamon has also shown signs of blocking the enzyme alanine, which allows the absorption of Glucose into the blood.

  - o **Fight Against Fungi and Bacteria:** Compounds found in cinnamon can help fight off bacteria and fungi. Test-tube research has shown that the main active component of cinnamon prevents the growth of bacteria and fungi, including Staphylococcus, Salmonella, and E.coli, which all cause illness in humans. The spice can also help avoid and treat Candida in the digestive tract. It can help with yeast growth which makes it a viable preventative supplement.

- **Anti-inflammatory Properties and Heart Health:** The antioxidants and polyphenols in cinnamon possess anti-inflammatory properties which can help fight chronic inflammation. It is particularly good for inflammation of the liver. Cinnamon contains heart-healthy compounds that may decrease inflammation and may help to raise levels of HDL (good) cholesterol. The spice may also help reduce blood pressure and LDL (bad) cholesterol levels. Cinnamon may also improve insulin resistance, blood glucose, and lipid metabolism; which help lower the risk of heart disease.

- **Defend Against Neurodegenerative Diseases:** Compounds in cinnamon may help stop the build-up of tau, a protein that is linked as a staple of Alzheimer's disease. Additionally, cinnamon helps improve motor functions, protect neurons, and normalizes neurotransmitter levels, all of which can aid in response to Parkinson's disease.

- **Dark Chocolate with Cocoa** – Quality dark chocolate is rich in iron, copper, manganese, and fiber. It can deliver antioxidants and minerals, which can positively affect health. However, it must be consumed in moderation as it may also contain high sugar and calories. Cocoa powder is made by crushing cocoa beans and removing the fat or cocoa butter. Although it is associated with making chocolate, some important compounds in cocoa can benefit health.

  - **Powerful Source of Antioxidants:** Cocoa is rich in polyphenols, flavanols, catechins, and many other organic compounds that biologically function as antioxidants. The polyphenols may help lower some forms of LDL (bad) cholesterol when combined with different foods like almonds and cocoa. Some studies have shown that cocoa and dark chocolate had more antioxidant activity than fruits tested, including blueberries and acai berries.

  - **Reduce Risk of Heart Disease:** The bio-compounds in cocoa may improve blood flow in the arteries and cause a small but statistically significant decrease in blood pressure. These compounds can aid in raising HDL (good) cholesterol and protect LDL (bad) cholesterol from oxidation. Research has shown a reduced risk for heart disease among those who consume moderate amounts of dark chocolate and cocoa.

- o **Improve Brain Function:** Cocoa or dark chocolate may improve brain function by increasing blood flow and supply to brain tissue. It also contains stimulants like caffeine and theobromine. Additionally, the Flavanols may support neuron production and brain function and may have a role in the prevention of age-related neurodegenerative diseases.

- o **Skin Health:** The flavanols in cocoa can help to protect the skin against sun damage, improve circulation and blood flow to the skin, and aid in increasing skin density and hydration.

- **Coffee** – While we know coffee is a boost of caffeine, it also contains antioxidants and over 100 biologically active compounds. These substances help reduce inflammation and oxidative stress, improve insulin sensitivity, boost metabolism, and may protect against disease. Aside from the soothing energy boost, the benefits of moderate consumption of coffee (1-2 cups per day) also include:

  - o **Living Longer:** Recent studies from Johns Hopkins University School of Medicine found that coffee drinkers are less likely to die from some of the leading causes of death in women, including coronary heart disease, stroke, diabetes, and kidney disease.

  - o **Process Glucose Better:** Some studies suggest that drinking coffee, whether caffeinated or decaffeinated, may reduce the risk of developing type 2 diabetes long term. Caffeine impairs glucose metabolism and insulin response in the short term, but many studies have found that long-term coffee consumption may lower the risk of developing type 2 diabetes. This is because coffee contains other compounds, such as chlorogenic acids (also found in fruits and vegetables), that may improve glucose metabolism in the long run.

  - o **Less Likely to Develop Heart Failure:** According to the American College of Cardiology, drinking two to three cups of coffee daily is associated with maintaining a healthy heart.

  - o **Less Likely to Develop Age-Related Neurological Disorders:** Coffee consumption has also been correlated with a decreased risk of developing neurodegenerative conditions like Alzheimer's disease and Parkinson's disease.

- o **Liver Health:** Some research studies show that regular coffee drinkers, of both regular and decaf, are more likely to have healthy liver enzyme levels in comparison to those who don't drink coffee regularly.

- o **Stronger DNA:** Dark roast coffee decreases breakage in DNA strands. This breakage in DNA strands occurs naturally but can lead to cancer or tumors if not repaired by the cells in the body.

- o **Lower Risk of Colon Cancer:** Researchers have found that coffee drinkers (regular & decaf) were 26% less likely to develop colon and rectal cancer.

- o **Less Likely to Suffer a Stroke:** It is recommended, especially for women, to drink at least one cup of coffee daily, as it is associated with lowered stroke risk. The fourth leading cause of death in women.

- **Fennel** – Fennel is a vegetable with a pale bulb, long green stems, and fronds. All parts of the fennel plant are edible. Yes, even the bulb and seeds! There are varieties of fennel treated as a vegetable and treated as an herb with foliage that resembles dill. It has a strong aniseed flavor making it a versatile ingredient. Fennel has a history of medicinal use for various respiratory, digestive, endocrine, and reproductive conditions. It is also used as a stimulant for lactating mothers. Studies also show that fennel contains health-protective antioxidants and antimicrobial, antiviral, anti-fungal, and anti-inflammatory compounds. Fennel is a good source of folate which is necessary for healthy red blood cell formulation. Including fennel and other folate-rich foods may improve the symptoms of anemia. Fennel is often used to help relax muscles and ease pain, and it has also been used as a sleep aid.

- **Fermented Foods** – Fermented foods, which were initially produced as a way to preserve food, may help increase both the shelf life and health benefits of many foods. The probiotic in fermented foods has been associated with improvement in digestion, immunity, weight loss, and more. Fermented food can also boost the number of beneficial or probiotics in the gut. Fermented foods or drinks that help boost digestion and overall health include:

  - o **Kefir:** Kefir is a fermented dairy product that may improve lactose digestion, decrease inflammation, and boost bone health.

  - o **Tempeh:** Tempeh is made from fermented soybeans. It is high in probiotics and may boost heart health. It is also a source of antioxidants.

- o **Natto:** Natto is also a fermented soybean product. It is high in fiber content and is known to promote bowel regularity. It has also been linked to preventing bone loss.

- o **Kombucha:** Kombucha is a fermented tea that can decrease blood sugar and reduce levels of cholesterol and triglycerides.

- o **Miso:** Miso is associated with improved heart health and reduces the risk of certain cancers, though more human studies are needed.

- o **Kimchi:** Kimchi is a Korean fermented food with properties that may help reduce insulin resistance and promote balanced cholesterol levels.

- o **Sauerkraut:** Sauerkraut is low in calories but contains plenty of fiber and Vitamins C and K. It is also packed with antioxidants important to the eyes.

- o **Probiotic Yogurt:** Probiotic yogurt has many nutrients and may help reduce body weight, lower blood pressure, and improve bone health.

- **Green Tea** – Green tea has been referred to as one of the healthiest beverages. It is loaded with antioxidants and has many potential health benefits.

  - o **Reduces Body Weight**: The polyphenols in green tea increase the body's rate of transforming food into calories.

  - o **Prevent Hair Loss:** The polyphenols and catechins block DHT, a hormone that is a driving force behind hair loss. Another component found in green tea, epigallocatechin gallate (EGCG), stimulates hair cell production and growth.

  - o **Fight Aging:** The polyphenols in green tea are potent antioxidants that may benefit and shield skin from harmful free radicals.

  - o **Lower Blood Pressure:** Green tea helps repress angiotensin, one cause of high blood pressure.

  - o **Encourages Oral Health:** Drinking green tea can lower the chance of cavities and other dental problems. Catechins and polyphenols are considered natural fluorides that kill bacteria that cause bad breath. Additionally, there is natural fluoride in green tea, which aids in preventing tooth decay.

- o **Makes Bones Strong:** The natural fluoride in green tea does more than aid dental health. It also contributes to bone density.

- o **Reduce the Risk of Cancer:** Antioxidants in green tea are so powerful that they may help lower the chance of cancer.

- o **Promote Longevity:** According to a Japanese study, people who consumed five or more cups of green tea per day were less likely to die within the 11-year testing period. Additionally, it was found to lower the risk of stroke and heart disease. Green tea contains high amounts of flavonoids and antioxidants linked to lower LDL cholesterol levels and improved cardiovascular health.

- o **Improve Brain Function:** Green tea could help protect the brain against two of the most common neurodegenerative disorders: Alzheimer's and Parkinson's.

- o **Lower Blood Sugar Levels:** The polyphenol and polysaccharide-rich tea leaves could help lower and stabilize blood sugar levels.

- **Himalayan Salt** – Pink Himalayan salt is a type of rock salt from the region of Pakistan. It contains sodium chloride, like table salt, but also has trace minerals such as potassium, magnesium, and calcium. This is what gives it the light pink tint. Replacing table salt with pink Himalayan salt can help lower sodium intake and increase intake of other rich minerals. Himalayan salt is a more natural salt and does not contain additives.

- **Lemongrass** – Lemongrass is a shrub-like herb commonly used in Southeast Asian cooking. The lower stalks and bulbs of the plant have a lemon scent and flavor often used to add flavor to teas, marinades, curries, and broths. In addition to being used as a flavoring agent while cooking, lemongrass and lemongrass essential oil have many medicinal purposes as well. Lemongrass has been linked with uses for treating Rheumatism, treating digestive tract spasms, achy joints, and vomiting. It has antibacterial properties and is often used as a mild astringent to kill germs. Other benefits linked to regular consumption of lemongrass or lemongrass oil include:

  - o Treat common cold symptoms: reducing fever, pain, swelling.

  - o Aid in improving sugar and cholesterol in the blood, which can also help reduce high blood pressure.

  - o In women, it can help stimulate the uterus and menstrual cycle.

- **Mint Tea** – Mint tea is an herbal tea made by steeping the leaves of plants in the mint family. Typically, mint tea is made from peppermint and spearmint leaves. Mint tea has been linked to benefiting digestion, and one of the most popular remedies for an upset stomach is to sip on a freshly brewed cup of peppermint tea.

    o **Soothe and Improve Digestive Systems:** The peppermint leaves contain compound essential oils, including menthol, menthone, and limonene; all of which can help to calm an upset stomach and aid with digestion. Peppermint oil has been shown to relax muscles in your digestive system and improve various digestive symptoms. Drinking peppermint tea can also ease irritable bowel syndrome (IBS) symptoms such as stomach pain, bloating, and flatulence. In fact, doctors often prescribe peppermint oil capsules as a remedy to help ease the symptoms of IBS. The mint helps the stomach muscles relax, improving the flow of bile through the system.

    o **Boost Mood and Mental Awareness:** The refreshing and stimulating effects of drinking mint tea are believed to help increase alertness and memory and improve concentration. The scent of peppermint stimulates the limbic system, which is what can make us more alert and improve focus.

    o **Natural Pain Remedy:** Mint tea's aroma positively affects the olfactory system. This could help ease tension headaches and migraines as the menthol oil vapors can help relax the tensed cranial muscles relieving the pain. Additionally, soothing compounds found in mint leaves are believed to help reduce the severity of menstrual cramping.

    o **Treat Bad Breath:** Peppermint oil has been shown to kill germs that lead to bad breath. This is why peppermint is a common ingredient in breath mints, chewing gum, and toothpaste. Mint tea is a flavorful and natural way to wash away bacteria in the mouth.

- **Moringa** – Moringa is a plant native to northern India but can also grow in other tropical and subtropical locations like Africa and Asia. The leaves, flowers, seeds, and roots have all been used in folk medicine for centuries. Moringa is a good source of vitamins B, C, D, and E. In fact, the leaves contain a high volume of Vitamin C and have been shown to contain more vitamin C than oranges.

Additionally, there is a high potassium content and a good source of calcium, protein, iron, zinc, and amino acids. These substances all help the body heal and build muscle. Moringa has been traditionally used to treat a wide range of conditions, including diabetes, infections (bacterial, viral, and fungal), joint pain, and heart health. Some health benefits of moringa include:

- o **Improved Eyesight:** Moringa contains eyesight-improving properties due to its high antioxidant levels. Moringa may stop the dilation of retinal vessels, help prevent the thickening of capillary membranes, and inhibit retinal dysfunction.

- o **Good for the Skin and Hair:** The abundance of antioxidants and nutrients in moringa leaves improves the health and appearance of skin and hair. The antioxidants in moringa leaves can reduce the appearance of fine lines and wrinkles on the skin. Moringa is also good for acne-prone skin. A paste of moringa leaves applied to the scalp and hair can help reduce dandruff and strengthen hair follicles.

- o **Lower Blood Sugar Levels:** Moringa leaves help to stabilize blood sugar levels due to the presence of isothiocyanates.

- **Nuts** – Nuts contain unsaturated fatty acids and other nutrients, making them a great snack food. Nuts inexpensive, easy to store, and easy to pack for on the go. Some nuts may be high in calories, so watch portions carefully! Research found that frequently eating nuts can help lower inflammation related to heart disease and diabetes. Nuts have also been linked to lowering the risk of blood clots.

- **Olive Oil** – Olive oil is produced through the natural crushing of olives and then refined without using solvents. It is high in heart-healthy monounsaturated fat and can be a source of antioxidants and polyphenols. It is one of the healthiest oils you can cook with. Nutrition experts believe the Mediterranean basin is home to some of the longest-living populations. They believe this is influenced by their typical daily diet, which is abundant in healthy fats from olive oil, nuts, and fatty fish.

In comparison to other cooking oils, olive oil has a unique potential to deliver compounds against degenerative diseases and chronic conditions due to its potent polyphenol compounds and the high percentage of monounsaturated fatty acids. As a result, regular consumption of olive oil has been associated with a wide range of health benefits from stronger bones to reduced pain and inflammation, as well as support for a healthy gut and immune system. Some studies link olive oil to improved memory, brain function, and cardiovascular health!

- o **Promotes Cardiovascular Health:** Studies have shown that people who ate a Mediterranean-style diet with extra virgin olive oil each day had a lower risk of developing cardiovascular disease. Additionally, it was shown that their risk of heart attack, stroke, and death from heart-related conditions was lower than those who consistently ate a low-fat diet. Consuming oleic acid-rich oils, which include olive oil, may reduce the risk of coronary heart disease.

- o **Improve Cholesterol and Blood Pressure Levels:** Olive oil has been linked to improved cholesterol levels and reduced blood pressure. This is thanks to oleic acid, abundant in olive oil, and the various polyphenols that work together to reduce inflammation and oxidative stress and affect the cholesterol levels in the bloodstream.

- o **Boost Memory, Brain, and Mental Health:** Polyphenols in olive oil (particularly the oleocanthal) are potent antioxidants that may help counter oxidative stress related to the progression of neurodegenerative diseases. Studies have shown that oleocanthal-rich olive oils help reduce neuro-inflammation and restore healthy blood-brain barrier functions, which could slow the progression of some neurodegenerative diseases. Research studies have linked olive oil' to support the central nervous system and improve nerve function. It is connected to increased levels of serotonin.

- o *ANCIENT FILIPINO SECRET #2:* Olive oil can be used as a moisturizer for the skin. I use olive oil as a moisturizer. I used coconut oil before, but now I prefer olive oil. I find olive oil to work better. It is my favorite moisturizer, from head to toe. It is better than the expensive moisturizers that I buy. I do still buy eye cream, retinol castor oil, and hydraulic acid to add to my olive oil. I still use coconut oil occasionally. For my veins, I crush bay leaves and put them in a bottle with olive oil to massage my legs. It helps, but my husband complains about the smell!

- **Rosemary leaves and tea-** Rosemary is an herb native to the Mediterranean region but is used in cooking all over the world. The rosemary leaves can be eaten fresh or dried, but it is most commonly used for tea or infused oil. Rosemary has a fresh but bitter taste and has many health benefits. The herb contains iron, potassium, calcium, and other essential minerals for good health. In natural medicine, rosemary has been believed to aid with stomach pain, bloating, and inflammation. It has also been known to improve circulation and boost the immune system. Rosemary leaves are a good source of antioxidant and anti-inflammatory compounds which may protect against some chronic diseases. Rosemary also has a high Manganese content. Manganese is an essential nutrient for metabolic health. The manganese also helps the body form blood clots allowing injuries to heal faster, making rosemary a natural remedy when injured. I use rosemary leaves faithfully in my daily smoothies. That must explain why I am healthy, happy, and content! It must also be why I am getting better and not older. What can I say?! Other health benefits of rosemary leaves and tea may include:

- **Reduce Stress and Improve Mood:** The anti-inflammatory and antioxidant properties make rosemary a natural choice for improving mood and memory. Researchers have also studied the effects of stress after drinking a cup of rosemary tea. The conclusion was that those who consumed the rosemary tea showed reduced stress levels and better moods after drinking the tea. Furthermore, rosemary has been linked with boosting the production of serotonin which also helps regulate mood and stress levels.

- **Support Vision and Eye Health:** Recent studies have shown that drinking rosemary tea can help reduce inflammation and improve blood flow to the eyes. One study showed that those who drink rosemary tea were less likely to develop age-related macular degeneration. The phytochemicals in rosemary may help improve eye health, and they can also help regulate liver function and lower the risk of asthma.

- **Support Brain Health:** Rosemary is rich in antioxidants which help protect the brain from damage. Studies found that people who drank rosemary tea regularly had improved performance on tests of short-term memory and problem-solving. Additionally, those who drank rosemary tea also had a reduced risk of developing diseases like Alzheimer's.

- **Reduced Risk of Cancer:** Rosemary leaves contain carnosic acid, a compound known for its powerful antioxidant properties. Carnosic acid can help to slow the growth of cancer cells and has even been shown to lower the risk of developing tumors.

Food and Inflammation

Inflammation is the body's normal response to illness and infection. There are several lines of defense which include white blood cells that attack intruders and antibodies that bind to them. There are a whole host of chemicals the body produces to fight off threats in the body - these are the inflammatory markers. Some forms of inflammation are visible. Symptoms usually include swelling, redness in the affected area, pain, and stiffness. A poor-quality diet can trigger low-level inflammation, which is not as visible. This is dangerous because diet-related inflammation is often undetected until it has already caused serious harm. The relationship with food can impact inflammation in the body. Some foods can cause inflammation, and some foods fight inflammation.

Foods That Increase Inflammation

When consumed regularly, some foods are more likely to result in obesity and cause nutrition-related chronic health conditions.

- **Foods with high added sugar** – Eating excessive added sugar can increase triglycerides, which may increase the risk of heart disease, tooth decay, and other chronic conditions.

- **Ultra-processed foods** – like most fast food and packaged snacks. If you read the label on a packaged snack and half of the ingredients are chemicals or words you don't know, don't buy it!

- **Dairy** – Many dairy foods have been deemed highly inflammatory due to the upset stomach, constipation, diarrhea, hives, and other issues it causes. Cheese, cream, and whole milk promote inflammation in the body, but plain yogurt may help reduce unpleasant inflammatory symptoms.

- **Fatty Red Meats** – Red meats like beef ribs, burgers, and ground beef cause inflammation due to the high bad-fat content. Bad fats include trans fats, saturated fat, hydrogenated fats, and oils. Excessive consumption of red meat may cause arthritis, especially inflammatory arthritis like gout.

- **Too many Omega-6 fatty acids** – Omega-6 fatty acids are essential for the body's overall health, but the body cannot make them. Omega-3 fatty acids and omega-6 fatty acids play a crucial role in brain function. They also play a critical role in growth and development. A healthy diet, however, contains a balance of mega-3 and omega-6 fatty acids. The omega-6 fatty acids tend to promote inflammation. The omega-3 fatty acids help to reduce inflammation.

- **Harmful Ingredients** – Generally, it is recommended to avoid foods high in harmful ingredients like high fructose corn syrup, color stabilizers and dyes, and corn sugar…to name a few.

- **Avoid gluten** – Studies have found that people with inflammation-related arthritis like rheumatoid arthritis and psoriatic arthritis may also have a higher risk for gluten intolerance.

The Top Anti-Inflammatory Foods

- **Nuts** – Walnuts, almonds, and many other nuts may help reduce inflammation and heart disease. Most nuts have a high "healthy" fat content as well as omega-3 fatty acids and fiber.

- **Celery** – Celery and celery seeds have around 25 anti-inflammatory compounds that can reduce inflammation and fight off infection. Celery contains substances that help blood pressure and strengthens resistance to heart disease.

- **Beets** – Beets are rich in fiber, folate, and plant pigments called betalains which have antioxidant and anti-inflammatory properties. Beets are rich in nitrates which reduce inflammation by removing harmful compounds from the bloodstream. Beets also contain magnesium which is essential to prevent the accumulation of calcium which can lead to kidney stones.

- **Broccoli** – Broccoli is rich in sulforaphane, an antioxidant that decreases inflammation by reducing the levels of cytokines and nuclear factor kappa B in the body. These are the molecules that drive inflammation in the body. Broccoli contains a very high amount of potassium and magnesium as well.

- **Pineapple** – The Bromelain in pineapple juice triggers the body's ability to reduce swelling and fight pain. It also helps fight off infection and lessens the risk of strokes and heart disease. Pineapple also supplies the daily dose of vitamin C and B-1.

- **Coconut Oil** – Coconut shows antioxidant activity due to its polyphenol content, and coconut oil is a rich source of phenolic compounds like caffeic acid, ferulic acid, and more. It is because of these polyphenols and their antioxidant properties they can help offset oxidative free radicals and are an effective anti-inflammatory.

- **Turmeric** - Research has shown that Turmeric reduces inflammation related to arthritis, diabetes, and other diseases. Turmeric's key element is Curcumin, a potent anti-inflammatory compound. Its role in treating rheumatoid arthritis shows how powerful it can be in the fight against inflammation.

- **Ginger** – Natural health experts claim that ginger helps lessen inflammation that occurs when the body's immune system malfunctions.

- **Blueberries and Many other Berries** – Berries contain antioxidants called anthocyanins. These compounds are what give berries anti-inflammatory properties. Additionally, eating blueberries may also help slow down the decline in mental abilities, and it may also help improve memory function.

- **Salmon** – Salmon, and many other fatty fish, are an excellent source of omega-3 fatty acids, eicosapentaenoic acid (EPA), and docosahexaenoic acid (DHA). The body metabolizes these fatty acids into compounds called resolvins and proteins, which also have anti-inflammatory effects.

Food and Diabetes

The Best Foods for People Living with Diabetes

- **Fatty Fish** – Fish like Salmon, Sardines, Anchovies, and Mackerel are great sources of omega-3 fatty acids, DHA and EPA, which have significant benefits for heart disease.

- **Leafy Greens** – Leafy greens have more vitamin C, which acts as a potent antioxidant and has anti-inflammatory qualities.

- **Avocados** – Avocados are a good source of healthy fat, fiber, and vitamins. They also contain antioxidants and anti-inflammatory compounds. The avocado's high potassium and magnesium content also helps keep blood pressure at healthy levels.

- **Eggs** – Eggs can help increase HDL (good) cholesterol levels and modify the size and shape of LDL (bad) cholesterol.

Foods and Habits that May Cause Diabetes

There are many diet habits you probably never knew could raise diabetic risk. If diabetes is a concern, foods, and routines to avoid include:

- **Eating Only Starchy Food** – It is best not to pair starchy vegetables with other carbohydrates—for example, rice with sweet potato.

- **Snacking on Dried Fruits** – Regular snacking on dried fruits can cause blood sugar spikes. Eating sparingly is okay.

- **Not Eat Enough Nuts and Seeds –** The healthy polyunsaturated fats found in nuts and seeds have been found to help prevent type 2 diabetes by improving insulin sensitivity.

- **Consuming Too Much Red Meat and Processed Meat –** Studies have shown red meat and processed meat like bacon and ham are all high in saturated fats. These saturated fats can raise blood sugar levels. Eating even a small portion of red meat on a frequent basis can increase the risk of diabetes. Also, try to avoid meat that has been overly-processed and is significantly beyond its native form.

- **Too Much Processed Food –** Overly processed foods typically contain a high volume of preservatives, chemicals, and sodium. Large quantities of these components are unsuitable for the body and can impact how the body processes needed nutrients.

Food and Acid Reflux

Acid reflux occurs when there is acid backflow from the stomach into the esophagus. The food consumed affects the amount of acid the stomach produces. Eating the right food is the key to controlling acid reflux or gastroesophageal reflux disease (GERD). GERD is a severe and chronic form of acid reflux.

Foods to Eat to Aid in Reducing Acid Reflux

- **Healthy Fats –** Reduce intake of saturated and trans fats. Replace them with unsaturated and healthy fats. Avocados, walnuts, flaxseed, and olive oil are all examples to increase consumption of healthy fats.

- **Egg Whites –** Egg whites have been linked to easing acid reflux, however, don't eat the yolks. Those are high in fat content, which can trigger acid reflux.

- **Ginger –** Ginger is naturally anti-inflammatory, which makes it a natural treatment for heartburn and other gastrointestinal conditions (cue the old ginger ale for upset stomach remedy!)

- **Oatmeal –** Oatmeal is high in fiber and a great way to absorb acid in the stomach. Diets high in fiber have been linked with a lower risk of acid reflux.

- **Fruits –** Non-citrus fruits are less likely to trigger acid reflux symptoms. Consider adding more melons, bananas, apples, or pears…but avoid adding more oranges, lemons, limes, or grapefruit.

- **Lean meat and seafood –** Lean meat such as chicken and turkey are great for reducing acid reflux when grilled, baked, or broiled - but not fried. Fish and seafood that are low-fat and high in fiber (like salmon) are a great source of protein that can reduce symptoms of acid reflux. Again, try these grilled, baked, broiled, or poached, but not fried.

Foods to Avoid or Eat Sparingly

- **Fried Foods** – Avoid fried and oily/greasy foods like french fries and onion rings. These foods can cause heartburn and acid reflux because they prevent the lower esophageal sphincter (LES) from tightening, allowing stomach acids to flow upward. Greasy foods are also harder to digest, so the stomach empties more slowly.

- **High-Fat Foods** – High-fat content can trigger acid reflux. Avoid full-fat dairy products like butter, whole milk, regular cheese, and sour cream. It is also best to avoid fatty cuts of beef, bacon fat, ham fat, and lard. Desserts, snacks, cream sauces, gravy, and salad dressings are also culprits of high-fat content.

- **Tomatoes and Citrus** – Highly acidic fruits and veggies like oranges, grapefruit, and tomatoes can cause or worsen acid reflux symptoms. Beware of foods that use these ingredients, especially tomatoes, like pizza sauce and salsa.

- **Chocolate** – Chocolate contains an ingredient called methylxanthine which has been shown to relax muscles in the LES, which can increase reflux.

- **Spicy or Tangy Foods** – Foods often used for flavoring like garlic, onions, and mint can often trigger heartburn and acid reflux.

Other Lifestyle Options

Other lifestyle habits that may also help reduce or relieve acid reflux symptoms include:

- Antacids and other medications can reduce acid production which may help with symptoms but, be aware, overuse can cause adverse side effects.

- Remain upright for at least 2 hours after eating. It is also best to eat slowly and avoid overeating.

- Avoid eating at least 3 to 4 hours before going to bed. Raising the head of the bed by 4 to 6 inches can help reduce symptoms while sleeping.

- Avoid alcohol and stop smoking.

Food and Heart Health

Heart disease is one of the leading causes of death in the United States. Lifestyle changes like reducing salt intake and getting more exercise have been proven to support heart health. What we eat can drastically affect our health. That said, the foods we include in our daily diet play a major role in lowering the risk for heart-related illnesses.

"Heart-Healthy" foods contain nutrients that can reduce the risk of heart disease by lowering the bad cholesterol (LDL), reducing blood pressure, improving insulin sensitivity, and more. On the other hand, there are a lot of foods that can negatively affect our heart health. So, what are the good and the bad? Some of these might surprise you!

Foods Known to Cause Heart Problems (According to cardiologists and dietitians)

- **Processed Deli Meat** – Cured deli meats contain preservatives called sodium nitrate. Nitrates have links to increasing internal inflammation. Chronic inflammation is directly linked to conditions affecting the arteries and heart health.

- Ketchup, Barbecue Sauce & "Reduced-Fat" Salad Dressings – These are culprits for hidden sodium and sugar content.

- **Fat-free Packaged Snacks** – These are also high in sodium and sugar.

- **Fancy Coffee Drinks** – These are high in sugar and fat.

- **Fruit Smoothies** – Serving size and sugar content are key. Smoothies can be healthy as long as they don't have too much in them. Think about how many pieces of fruit it takes to make that delicious smoothie. Then pack on the grams of sugar for additions like yogurt. Furthermore, drinking fruit instead of eating it whole reduces the fiber gained from the fruit.

- **White Bread and White Rice** – These are overly processed and are quite harmful to the heart.

- **Energy Drinks and Sports Drinks** – These drinks are jammed with sugar. Energy drinks are also a surge of caffeine that can cause unnecessary stress on the heart.

- **Diet Sodas** – While diet sodas may not have sugar or calories, they are full of artificial sweeteners. Long-term or daily intake of artificial sweeteners are linked to a higher risk of stroke, heart disease, and overall death.

- **Alcohol** – Excessive or regular alcohol consumption often leads to weight gain, a factor linked to developing high blood pressure and heart disease.

Foods for a Healthy Heart

- **Salmon & Sardines** – (Noticing a trend yet?) The omega-3 fatty acids in salmon and sardines improve metabolic markers for heart disease. Salmon has a high level of selenium, an antioxidant shown to improve cardiovascular protection. Sardines provide omega-3s in the form of fish oil which increases good cholesterol levels and reduces the risk of sudden heart attack, even in people who have had previous attacks.

- **Walnuts and Almonds** – These are good sources of omega-3 fatty acids. Nuts are also a good source of fiber and folate.

- **Chia Seeds** – A spoonful of chia seeds is low-calorie while providing a plant-based source of omega-3 fatty acids that help reduce bad cholesterol and plaque build-up.

- **Red Wine** – Some researchers suggest drinking moderate amounts of wine can improve heart health. Resveratrol, a compound with antioxidant properties, is found in dark-skinned berries and grapes. This antioxidant has also been linked with preventing cancer. Furthermore, red wines typically contain large amounts of procyanidins, an antioxidant that helps reduce cholesterol and improve the health of the arteries.

- **Brussel Sprouts** – The benefits of Brussel sprouts include reducing inflammation in the cardiovascular system and improving blood vessel health.

- **Oranges** – Oranges are a source of pectin, which blocks the absorption of cholesterol. They also contain a flavonoid that reduces inflammation of the arteries and lowers blood pressure. The citrus in oranges contains hesperidin, which helps improve blood flow to the heart, and Vitamin C, which is linked to protecting against stroke.

CHAPTER XV:
Supplements

Anti-Aging Supplements

While we can't stop ourselves from aging, we can make dietary and lifestyle changes to help slow some aging processes. The leading cause of aging includes accumulated cellular damage. This damage is caused by reactive molecules called free radicals. Following a nutrient-rich diet and exercising regularly can support healthy aging, but there are also supplements that may help with slowing the aging process.

Anti-Aging Vitamins and Supplements

- **Collagen** – As we age, the production of collagen, a protein that helps maintain skin structure, slows down, which leads to accelerated signs of aging.

- **CoQ10** – Coenzyme Q10 (CoQ10) is an antioxidant that the body produces. It plays an essential role in energy production and protects against cellular damage.

- **EGCG** – Epigallocatechin gallate (EGCG) is a well-known polyphenol compound in green tea. It offers impressive health benefits, including a reduced risk of certain cancers and heart disease. (I don't take any supplements; I just drink green tea regularly.)

- **Vitamin C** – Vitamin C is a powerful antioxidant in the body. It helps protect cells from oxidative damage.

- **Curcumin** – The main active compound in Turmeric. It has been shown to possess powerful cellular protective properties. It may help to slow aging by activating specific proteins and can protect against cellular damage.

There are many vitamins and supplements that may support healthy aging; however, more human research is needed. Some of these include:

- **Vitamin E** – Research suggests vitamin E has important roles in immune function and regulation of inflammation. Some studies have shown that older adults may need more of this vitamin to maintain health during the aging process.

- **Resveratrol** – An antioxidant found in grapes, peanuts, and red wine that activates enzymes called sirtuins and may promote longevity.

- **Sulforaphane** – A compound packed in cruciferous vegetables, like broccoli, known to have potent anti-inflammatory properties. Sulforaphane has been shown to reduce cancer cell ability to multiply. Which means it may slow the spread of cancer or slow tumor growth.

- **Vitamins K2 and D3** – One of the main functions of Vitamin K2 and D is reducing inflammation, which keeps the blood flowing to and from the heart properly. These vitamins can also aid with digestive problems, acid reflux, arterial plaques, depression, and even weak teeth or bones.

My Personal Supplements

Daily Morning Supplements

- Multi-vitamin supplement
- Vitamin B-12
- Kelp
- Biotin
- Vitamin D3
- Brewer's Yeast

Daily Evening Supplements

- Potassium
- Magnesium
- CoQ10
- Collagen

I am taking vitamin D3 supplements but only eating foods with K2 nutrients. These are hard cheese, soft cheese, egg yolk, and curd cheese. Other sources of K2 are natto goose liver, goose leaf, butter, and chicken liver. This is the reason why I am not afraid of dairy! I learned about K2 a long time ago.

In my daily food intake, I make sure to include the following:

- Rosemary leaves
- Cocoa
- Olive Oil
- Chia Seeds
- Himalayan salt
- Non-fat Greek Yogurt
- Hard and soft cheese
- Cinnamon
- Green Leafy vegetables
- In-season fruit and veggie

CHAPTER XVI:
Recipes

JUICE or SMOOTHIE RECIPES

Add ice and blend to make any of these juices into a smoothie.

Celery and Pineapple Juice

- 2 tsp ACV
- 2 stalks of celery
- 2 tsp rosemary
- ½ bunch cilantro
- 2 slices of pineapple
- ¼ tsp pink Himalayan salt
- 1 tsp cinnamon

Triple Berry Juice

- 1 cup frozen mixed berries
- 1 lemon
- ½ tsp pink Himalayan salt
- 2 tsp ACV
- 1 tsp cinnamon
- 2 stalks of celery
- Sprinkle of rosemary leaves
- 1 tsp chia seeds

Greens Juice
Makes 3-4 servings.

- 4 leaves of Kale
- 2 limes
- 1 tsp pink Himalayan salt
- 4 stalks of celery
- 2 large oranges
- 2 cloves
- ½ bunch of cilantro
- ½ cup of water

DIP & SALAD DRESSING

Blue Cheese & Yogurt Dip

- 8 oz. non-fat plain Greek yogurt
- 5 oz. of blue cheese
- dash of black and/or red pepper

For Salad:
- Salad Greens
- Olives
- Shredded or chopped carrots
- Optional: Choice of Nuts

Mix yogurt, blue cheese, and black or red pepper. Use it as a dip with your favorite veggies. You can also use this as a salad dressing on your choice of salad greens. Add some olives and carrots on top and enjoy!

SOUPS

Beef Vegetable Soup

- 1-2 lbs. lean beef
- 3 carrots
- 1 whole onion
- 1 turnip
- 5-6 cups of water
- ½ bunch of parsley
- 2 tsp pink Himalayan salt
- 1 bell pepper

Start by chopping your beef into cubes, cutting up all vegetables, and putting them into a large pot. Add water and salt and bring to a boil. Turn down the heat, cover, and simmer until all vegetables are soft. Be careful not to overcook.

Tip: You can also brown your beef cubes in a skillet with olive oil before adding them to the pot for added flavor.

Chicken Soup

- 1 lb. skinless chicken legs
- 2 cut-up green onions
- 1 bell pepper
- 3 carrots
- 2 tsp pink Himalayan salt
- 1 chopped onion
- 2 stalks of celery
- 4-5 cups of water

For this, you can use fresh or frozen chicken. Start by chopping up all your veggies and set them aside.

Add the onion, chicken, and pink Himalayan salt to a large pot. Boil until the chicken is cooked through. Add the carrots and simmer for 10 minutes. Then add the bell pepper and celery. Flake the chicken and throw it back in the pot. Give it a good stir and let simmer until the remaining veggies reach desired softness. Sprinkle with green onion and enjoy!

Sinigang (Filipino Sour Soup)

- 1 - 2 lbs. of lean beef, pork, or chicken
- 1 bunch of spinach
- 6-8 lemons, juiced
- 1 tsp. Pink Himalayan Salt
- 1 onion, chopped
- 1 clove of garlic
- 4-6 cups of water

Start by cubing up your choice of meat and finely chop garlic cloves. Lightly sauté the garlic, then add the chopped onion, salt, and lemon juice. Add your choice of meat and cook until brown. Add the water and bring it to a boil. Then reduce heat and simmer until the meat is tender. Once the meat is cooked through, add the spinach (you can add any of your favorite veggies if you wish). Let sit until the spinach is soft. Serve hot.

Other veggies that go well with Sinigang are okra and tomatoes; if you like it spicy, add some hot peppers. You can also use unripe tamarind in place of lemon for the souring agent.

MAIN DISH ENTREES

Broiled Chicken

- Pink Himalayan salt
- Olive oil
- Rosemary leaves
- Black pepper
- Whole Chicken

Preheat the oven to a broiler temperature of 375 degrees. Cut your chicken in half lengthwise. Wash under running water and drain. Remove the fat and skin. Place in your baking dish. Brush with olive oil and sprinkle with Rosemary leaves. Add salt and pepper to your liking. Broil until brown. Turn the chicken over and turn off the heat. Leave the chicken for 10 to 20 more minutes.

Beef & Broccoli

- 1 cup broccoli florets
- 1 lb. sirloin
- 3 tsp cornstarch
- 1 onion
- 1 tsp pink Himalayan salt
- 2 tbsp low sodium soy sauce
- ½ to 1 cup water
- 2 tsp olive oil

Cut the beef and onions julienne style. Heat the pan and olive oil, then fry the beef until brown. Sprinkle in the salt. Add the onion and wait until cooked. Then add the broccoli. Mix the soy sauce, water, and cornstarch in a separate container or bowl. Once it looks smooth, pour it into the pan. Serve hot.

Philippines Beef Steak

- 2 lbs. lean beef
- 4 lemons
- 1 onion
- low sodium soy sauce
- 1 green onion
- ¼ tsp pepper

PREP: Slice beef into strips. Marinate in soy sauce, squeeze the lemons over the meat and soy sauce (Tip: Watch for seeds, use a small strainer to catch seeds!), and add pepper. Mix well, and make sure all the meat is covered with the mixture. Marinate for at least two hours.

COOK: Slice the onion into rings and set aside. Heat a large frying pan and add the olive oil. Drain your beef but save the juice for later. Stir fry the beef until cooked on both sides. Pour the marinated juice over the meat. Cover and let it simmer for 15 minutes or until the meat is tender. Add the onion. Turn off the stove and let simmer/onions soften. Serve while hot.

Philippines Chop Suey

- 2 skinless chicken breasts
- 1 whole green pepper
- handful of fresh green beans
- 2 carrots
- 8 oz. fresh mushrooms
- ½ bunch of green onions
- 2 tsp red pepper
- ½ bunch of parsley
- Bean sprouts (optional)
- 2 tsp Olive Oil
- ½ tsp pink Himalayan salt
- 2 tsp corn-starch
- 4 cups of water

Boil the water, pink Himalayan salt, and chicken breast for 15 minutes. Set the chicken stock aside. Cut the vegetables julienne style and slice the chicken. Fry the sliced chicken with olive oil until it's stir-fried. Add the carrots and stir fry until tender. Add the green beans to fry for a minute, then add the chicken stock. Add the remaining vegetables except for the green onions and parsley. Then add the water to the cornstarch -- stir until it is smooth. Pour into the pan and stir. Turn off the stove and add the green onion and parsley. Serve hot.

Grilled Salmon

- 2 tsp. Rosemary leaves
- 2 tsp olive oil
- ¼ clove of garlic

- Dash of Pink Himalayan salt
- Dash of red pepper

Sprinkle the spices on the salmon. Heat the grill or iron pan. Put oil in the iron pan. If using the grill, pour the oil onto the fish and pat it. Cook in an iron pan or on the grill until the outside is crispy. Turn the fish over and cook the other side. Put on a plate with paper towels at the bottom. Take the paper towel out and transfer it to a different dish. Serve hot with your favorite veggies.

VEGETABLES

Kale With Egg Sauce
Makes 1 Serving

- 1 cup kale, chopped
- 2 hard-cooked eggs
- ½ cup water
- 2 tbsp prepared mustard
- ½ tsp pink Himalayan salt
- 2 tsp Apple Cider Vinegar

Combine the salt, chopped kale, and water in a saucepan. Cover and simmer over moderate heat. Peel the hard-cooked eggs and separate the yolks from the egg whites. Mash the yolk and stir in prepared mustard and apple cider vinegar. Drain the cooked kale and add the yolk mixture to the kale. Garnish with the cooked egg whites.

Green Beans in Vinaigrette
Makes 1 Serving

- ¾ lb. of green beans
- 1 tsp green onion
- ¼ cup of water
- Pinch of Pink Himalayan salt
- 1 tsp Apple Cider Vinegar
- 1 tsp olive oil

Cut green beans julienne style. Combine green beans, water, and Himalayan salt in a saucepan. Cover, and simmer over moderate heat, stirring occasionally. Drain excess liquid. Stir in Apple Cider Vinegar, olive oil, and chopped green onions.

Filipino Cabbage
Makes 1 Serving

- 1 qt. shredded Napa cabbage
- 1.5 tsp red or black pepper
- ½ cup diagonally sliced celery
- ⅓ cup green onion
- ¾ cup green pepper, thinly sliced
- Pinch of Pink Himalayan salt
- 2-3 spoons of olive oil

Heat olive oil in a saucepan. Add napa cabbage, celery, and green pepper. Add salt and pepper to taste. Cook on moderate heat until the cabbage is wilted. Add chopped green onions before serving.

Bok Choy (Chinese Chard)
Makes 1 Serving

- 1 cup Bok Choy thinly sliced
- Dash of powdered ginger
- 2 tsp. Cornstarch
- 3 tsp water
- 1 tsp low sodium soy sauce
- ¼ tsp pink Himalayan salt
- 1 tsp olive oil

Heat olive oil in a saucepan, and add Bok Choy, ginger, and salt. Combine soy sauce, water, and cornstarch. Stir well. Pour into the pan, stirring occasionally. Do not overcook.

DESSERTS

Carrot Delight
Makes 1 Serving

- 2 cups shredded carrots
- 8 oz. plain Greek yogurt
- Optional: a handful of dates

Mix carrots, dates, and yogurt in a mixing bowl. Refrigerate. Serve cold.

Creamy Apples
Makes 1-2 Servings

- 2 tsp. Apple Cider Vinegar
- 8 oz. Non-fat Greek yogurt
- Cinnamon
- 1-2 chopped apples

Mix chopped apples, apple cider vinegar, and yogurt. Add cinnamon to taste, and enjoy!

Creamy Pineapples
Makes 1-2 Servings

- 2 tsp. Apple Cider Vinegar
- 8 oz. Non-fat Greek yogurt
- Cinnamon
- Chopped fresh pineapple

Mix chopped pineapples, apple cider vinegar, and yogurt together. Add cinnamon to taste, and enjoy!

CONCLUSION

In part three, we covered what to be aware of and what our body needs and doesn't need. Our bodies need nutrients to do what we need to do and think well. We need nutrients like good fats and food rich in vitamins, antioxidants, protein, and fiber. We get these nutrients with a well-balanced diet that includes fresh fruit and vegetables, lean meats, and protein.

Sticking with natural food may promote health and wellness. Nutritious food is essential to healthy living. I included some supplements, nutritious food, and recipes I found helpful to my healthy living.

What our body doesn't need are chemicals, pesticides, too many carbs, bad oil, preservatives, and simply just too much food. Everything in moderation. Frustration and disappointment are part of our daily lives. Our reaction toward these obstacles will significantly impact our mental health. Being mindful and aware of how our mind affects our bodies can improve our health and cognitive function. Mental clarity and function will help us avoid eating junk food to make us feel better because we are aware that it is a part of life and can handle it.

My family suffering and dying from diabetes inspired me to write this book. My research and interest in good health have helped me in many ways. I can think positively. I make better choices and decisions because of my healthy habits. It helped me pay attention to what I eat, when, and how much I eat. Choosing higher fiber helps digestion. Supplements supply the nutrients that are lacking in my diet. Keeping an eye on the bad fats has slimmed me down. Incorporating good fats such as MCT oil, olive oil, and Omega-3 have been good additions to my diet. Learning about food has helped me meet my health goals. Whole food, plant-based and natural foods are my best choice for eating healthy.

Moving and exercising may help reduce the risk of diabetes and other illnesses. Exercise may reduce depression, type 2 diabetes, heart disease, and more. We should not be lazy but, instead, do something easy. Start small, and tomorrow do a little more. Then the next day, a little bit more. Before we know it, we will be accomplishing much more than we realize. Being overweight or obese may lead to diabetes and other health problems, but being underweight may also affect overall health.

Water is necessary to be healthy. It keeps us hydrated, helps digestion, and detoxifies our system by moving toxins through our kidneys. Stay hydrated. Dehydration leads to health problems. Health problems may also cause dehydration. We must stay hydrated at all times for optimal health. Our body functions better when we are hydrated. Our skin will look fresh, soft, and clear. Dehydration will cause wrinkles and rashes. Staying hydrated may also aid in weight loss. Water has no calories, and it can help aid satiation. Drinking water may also boost energy and digestion.

Sleep and relaxation will help control our behavior and emotions. How we feel while awake depends on how much rest and sleep we had the night before and will get that evening. Lack of sleep has been linked to diabetes, heart problems, and stroke. Sleep deprivation can affect our appearance. Lack of sleep means more wrinkles.

Manufacturers add chemicals to make food taste better and last longer. These are additives, preservatives, processed foods, hydrogenated oils, and more. These harmful ingredients will make us ill slowly. Don't be one who doesn't pay attention until it is too late. Then, it is hard to change. Our body needs natural foods, whole foods, and nutritious food. Taking supplements may help provide the nutrients lacking in our diet. Eating unhealthy food affects our mood, our health, and our brain.

Optimal health is living your best life. It is different for everybody. My best life may not be your best life. Stress will destroy optimal health. Simple living may eliminate some of the unnecessary stress. Meditation, praying, walking, enjoying the sun, practicing deep breathing, and relaxing are all ways to achieve the best life. Everyone has different ways of staying fit and handling stress. Doing the best we know is the way to go. Just take it easy and enjoy life.

We can have the life we want. We must know what that is and go after it. People don't get what they want in life because they often don't know what it is that they want. The final ancient secret came from my hero, my dad. He encouraged us to live simply and humbly. He always said, "Living nobly and humbly is where true happiness comes from. It is the key to a happy and healthy life." When we don't know what we want, we should start with a humble beginning and ask God. If we believe, with God's help, we will get what we want. I am thankful for everything that happens, knowing they are from God. When things don't go the way I want, I know God is stopping me from ruining my life. I genuinely believe that.

"⁵Trust in the LORD with all your heart and lean not on your own understanding. ⁶ In all your ways submit to HIM, and he will make your path." - Proverbs 3:5-6

This was an epic journey. Thank you for reading and joining me in my journey to write this book. Fill your heart with joy and laughter. May you have the best days ahead of you. Wishing you success in the years to come. Always remember, "Health is wealth." Now let's take care of each other.

GLOSSARY

Adrenaline - Hormone secreted by the adrenal glands, especially in conditions of stress, increasing rates of blood circulation, breathing, carbohydrate metabolism prepares muscles for exertion.

Apple Cider Vinegar (ACV) - A vinegar, or cider vinegar, made from fermented apple juice, and used in salad dressing, marinades, vinaigrettes, food preservatives, and chutneys. It is made by crushing apples, then squeezing out the juice.

Advanced Glycation End products (AGEs) - Proteins or lipids that become glycated after exposure to sugars. AGEs are prevalent in diabetic vasculature and contribute to development of atherosclerosis.

Alzheimer's disease - A progressive disease that destroys memory and other important mental functions.

Anti-inflammatory - Characterization for substances that aid in fighting inflammation.

Angiotensin - A protein whose presence in the blood promotes aldosterone secretion and tends to raise blood pressures.

Anthocyanin - Colored, water-soluble pigments that belong to the phenolic group. Depending on their pH may appear red, blue, or black.

Atherosclerosis - Disease of arteries characterized by disposition of plaques of fatty material on their inner walls.

Arthritis - Chronic inflammation affecting many joints.

Carotenoids - Any of a class of mainly yellow, orange, or red fat-soluble pigments that give color to plants.

Casein - The main protein present in milk, and cheese

Catechin - Main substance found in tea that helps to protect cells from damage caused by free radicals.

Colorectal cancer - Cancer of the colon or rectum.

Cortisol - The primary stress hormone, increases sugar in the bloodstream, enhances the brain's use of glucose.

C-Reactive Protein (CRP) - A protein made in the liver and released into the bloodstream, usually in low concentrations. The liver releases more CRP into the bloodstream if there is inflammation in the body. High levels of CRP may indicate a serious health condition that causes inflammation.

Diabetes - A disease in which the body's ability to produce or respond to the hormone insulin is impaired, resulting in abnormal metabolism of carbohydrates and elevated levels of glucose in the blood and urine.

Endorphins - Any of the group of hormones secreted within the brain and nervous system and having several physiological functions. They are peptides which activate the body's opiate receptors, and cause an analgesic, or drug-like, effect.

Gastrointestinal - Relating to the stomach and/or intestines.

Ghrelin -The "hunger hormone." This hormone is produced by the stomach and released to signal to the brain when the stomach is empty, and it is time to eat.

Glutathione - A substance made from amino acids glycine, cysteine, and glutamic acid. It is produced by the liver and involved in many of the body's processes. Glutathione is used in tissue building and repair as well as immune system function.

Hydrogenated - The process in which a liquid oil changes into a solid.

Hydroxytyrosol - A phenolic compound found in olive oils and wines. Considered a powerful antioxidant with anti-inflammatory benefits and protector of the skin and eyes.

Inflammation - A localized physical condition where a part of the body becomes reddened, swollen, hot and often painful.

Usually, part of the body's reaction to injury or infection.

Insomnia - A common sleep disorder that can make it hard to fall asleep, hard to stay asleep, or cause a person to wake up too early and not be able to get back to sleep.

Iron - An important mineral for making red blood cells which carry oxygen around the body. A lack of iron can lead to anemia. The iron needed should be received from a balanced daily diet, but it is also available as a supplement.

Leptin - A hormone that the adipose tissue (body fat) releases to help the body maintain normal weight on a long-term basis. It is also known as an appetite suppressant.

Lipoprotein - Protein that are combine with and transport fat or other lipids in blood plasma.

Luteolin - A flavonoid with potential for cancer prevention and therapy. It is a yellow crystal in pure form and is food-derived typically present in glycosylated form in celery, green pepper and chamomile tea.

Melatonin - A hormone the brain produces in response to darkness. It helps control the body's sleep cycle, and it is an antioxidant. Also sold as a supplement.

Neurodegenerative - Characterized by degeneration of the nervous system, especially the neurons in the brain.

Nicotinamide - A water-soluble form of vitamin B3 or niacin. It is made in the body when consuming niacin-rich foods like fish, poultry, and nuts. Nicotinamide supplements are used to treat skin conditions and niacin deficiencies.

Oleic Acid - A fatty acid that occurs naturally in various animal and vegetable fats and oils. It is used for preventing heart disease and reducing cholesterol.

Polyphenols - A class of compounds found in plant foods that includes flavonoids, phenolic acids, lignans, and stilbenes. There are more than 8,000 different types of polyphenols that have been identified. Most polyphenols work as antioxidants in the body.

INDEX

REFERENCES

Pritzker , S. (2022, October 23). *Blue Cheese Nutrition Facts and Health Benefits*. Verywell Fit. Retrieved November 2022, from https://www.verywellfit.com/blue-cheese-nutrition-facts-and-health-benefits-5206366

10 heart-healthy foods that also taste awesome. Men's Health. (2023, February 6). Retrieved February 16, 2023, from https://www.menshealth.com/nutrition/g34641676/best-heart-healthy-foods/

12 health benefits of Chia seeds. Facty. (2021, January 20). Retrieved December 2022, from https://facty.com/food/nutrition/13-health-benefits-of-chia-seeds/

5 reasons why believing is important. Work hard play harderblog. (2017, November 17). Retrieved 2022, from https://workhardplayharder.blog/why-believing-is-important/

5 tips for creating belief. Work hard play harderblog. (2017, November 25). Retrieved 2022, from https://workhardplayharder.blog/5-tips-for-creating-belief/

9 reasons why (the right amount of) coffee is good for you. 9 Reasons Why (the Right Amount of) Coffee Is Good for You | Johns Hopkins Medicine. (2021, October 28). Retrieved December 2022, from https://www.hopkinsmedicine.org/health/wellness-and-prevention/9-reasons-why-the-right-amount-of-coffee-is-good-for-you

Amaresan, S. (2021, April 29). *10 creative ways to keep a positive attitude no matter what*. HubSpot Blog. Retrieved 2022, from https://blog.hubspot.com/service/positive-attitude

Benefit from sleep. Sleep is good medicine. (2022, July 25). Retrieved 2022, from https://sleepisgoodmedicine.com/benefit-from-sleep/

Bennett, C. (2019, November 26). *The health benefits of CILANTRO (coriander)*. News. Retrieved 2022, from https://www.news-medical.net/health/The-Health-Benefits-of-Cilantro-(Coriander).aspx

The best teas to help you sleep. Sleep Foundation. (2022, April 11). Retrieved 2022, from https://www.sleepfoundation.org/best-tea-for-sleep

Bolen, B. (2022, August 31). *The benefits of magnesium*. Verywell Health. Retrieved 2022, from https://www.verywellhealth.com/magnesium-for-constipation-and-ibsc-1944780

Burch, K. (2021, June 11). *CBD for diabetes*. Verywell Health. Retrieved 2022, from https://www.verywellhealth.com/cbd-oil-for-diabetes-5113061

Cardiomyopathy. www.heart.org. (n.d.). Retrieved 2022, from
https://www.heart.org/en/health-topics/cardiomyopathy

Christian, L. (2021, July 13). *How to believe in yourself (in 5 simple steps)*. SoulSalt.
Retrieved 2022, from https://soulsalt.com/how-to-believe-in-yourself/

A closer look at good cholesterol. Harvard Health. (2022, March 1). Retrieved 2022, from
https://www.health.harvard.edu/staying-healthy/a-closer-look-at-good-
cholesterol

Cuncic, A. (n.d.). *6 ways to deal with negative thoughts*. Verywell Mind. Retrieved 2022,
from https://www.verywellmind.com/how-to-change-negative-thinking-
3024843

The difference between health and wellness: Article: Sanford Wellness. Article | Sanford
Wellness. (n.d.). Retrieved 2022, from
https://occmed.sanfordhealth.org/resources/article-library/the-difference-
between-health-and-wellness

Encyclopædia Britannica, inc. (1998, July 20). *Cognition*. Encyclopædia Britannica.
Retrieved 2022, from https://www.britannica.com/topic/cognition-thought-
process

Happiness. Vocabulary.com. (n.d.). Retrieved 2022, from
https://www.vocabulary.com/dictionary/happiness

Harvard Health. (n.d.). Retrieved 2022, from
https://www.health.harvard.edu/topics/exercise-and-fitness#exercise-fitness3

How to create a positive mindset and attitude in life. Intelligent Change. (n.d.). Retrieved
2022, from https://www.intelligentchange.com/blogs/read/how-to-create-
positive-mindset-and-attitude

The link between nutrition and sleep. National Sleep Foundation. (2020, November 12).
Retrieved 2022, from https://www.thensf.org/the-link-between-nutrition-and-
sleep/

Maloney, B. (2022, November 8). *The effects of negativity*. Marque Medical. Retrieved
December 2022, from https://marquemedical.com/effects-of-negativity/

Mayo Foundation for Medical Education and Research. (2020, April). *Diabetic
neuropathy*. Mayo Clinic. Retrieved 2022, from
https://www.mayoclinic.org/diseases-conditions/diabetic-
neuropathy/symptoms-causes/syc-
20371580#:~:text=Peripheral%20neuropathy&text=It%27s%20the%20most%20c
ommon%20type,feel%20pain%20or%20temperature%20changes

Mayo Foundation for Medical Education and Research. (2022, August 3). *Exercise and
stress: Get moving to manage stress*. Mayo Clinic. Retrieved 2022, from

https://www.mayoclinic.org/healthy-lifestyle/stress-management/in-depth/exercise-and-stress

Mayo Foundation for Medical Education and Research. (2022, February 3). *How to stop negative self-talk.* Mayo Clinic. Retrieved February 2022, from https://www.mayoclinic.org/healthy-lifestyle/stress-management/in-depth/positive-thinking/art-20043950

MediLexicon International. (n.d.). *Moringa: Benefits, side effects, and risks.* Medical News Today. Retrieved 2022, from https://www.medicalnewstoday.com/articles/319916#what-is-in-moringa

Panoff, L. (2019, November 7). *6 benefits and uses of Rosemary Tea.* Healthline. Retrieved 2022, from https://www.healthline.com/nutrition/rosemary-tea

Self-Care - What is Self-Care? The University of Toledo. (n.d.). Retrieved 2022, from https://www.utoledo.edu/studentaffairs/counseling/selfhelp/copingskills/selfcare.html

Semeco, A. (2021, December 14). *Exercise: The top 10 benefits of regular physical activity.* Healthline. Retrieved February 2022, from https://www.healthline.com/nutrition/10-benefits-of-exercise#TOC_TITLE_HDR_6

SHFAustralia. (2020, June 23). *Caffeine, food, alcohol, smoking and sleep.* The Sleep Health Foundation. Retrieved 2022, from https://www.sleephealthfoundation.org.au/caffeine-food-alcohol-smoking-and-sleep.html

Spritzler, F. (2019, April 24). *11 reasons why berries are among the healthiest foods on Earth.* Healthline. Retrieved February 2022, from https://www.healthline.com/nutrition/11-reasons-to-eat-berries

Stibich, M. (n.d.). *10 top health benefits of sleep.* Verywell Health. Retrieved 2022, from https://www.verywellhealth.com/top-health-benefits-of-a-good-nights-sleep-2223766

Sumner, A. (2020, March 14). *Salute the sunshine: The healing power of the sun.* WellBeing Magazine. Retrieved 2022, from https://www.wellbeing.com.au/body/health/salute-sunshine-healing-power-sun.html

Type 1 diabetes self-care manual. Type 1 Diabetes Self-Care Manual | ADA. (n.d.). Retrieved 2022, from https://diabetes.org/diabetes/type-1/type-1-self-care-manual

Walsh, K. (2022, August). *These sneaky foods could be damaging your heart.* Prevention. Retrieved 2022, from https://www.prevention.com/health/health-conditions/g26221895/worst-foods-heart-health/

What does self-care mean for individuals with diabetes? USC. (2018, January 9). Retrieved April 2022, from https://nursing.usc.edu/blog/self-care-with-diabetes/

What exercises are best for heart health? Harvard Health. (n.d.). Retrieved 2022, from https://www.health.harvard.edu/topics/exercise-and-fitness#exercise-fitness5

What is diabetes? www.heart.org. (2022, July 12). Retrieved January 2023, from https://www.heart.org/en/health-topics/diabetes/about-diabetes

Wicks, L. (n.d.). *6 amazing health benefits of carrots.* EatingWell. Retrieved 2022, from https://www.eatingwell.com/article/2060606/health-benefits-of-carrots

Widener, C. (2017, February 8). *7 steps to achieve your dream.* SUCCESS. Retrieved 2022, from https://www.success.com/7-steps-to-achieve-your-dream/

Wilkinson, M. (2011, October 18). *Why do you need a plan?* Management Library. Retrieved 2022, from https://management.org/blogs/strategic-planning/2013/04/17/why-do-you-need-a-plan/

Yugay, I. (2018, January 10). *Why praising yourself is the recipe for self-confidence.* Mindvalley Blog. Retrieved 2022, from https://blog.mindvalley.com/self-confidence-and-praising/